Nielsen
450 Drehner
St Louis Mo
63132

THERAPEUTIC EXERCISE

(Second Edition)

THERAPEUTIC EXERCISE

By

HANS KRAUS, M.D.

*Associate Clinical Professor of
Rehabilitation and Physical Medicine
New York University College of Medicine*

Illustrations by

RICHARD KROTH

and

MADI KRAUS

With a Foreword by

HOWARD A. RUSK, M.D.

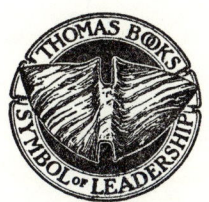

CHARLES C THOMAS • PUBLISHER
Springfield • *Illinois* • *U.S.A.*

Published and Distributed Throughout the World by

CHARLES C THOMAS • PUBLISHER
BANNERSTONE HOUSE
301-327 East Lawrence Avenue, Springfield, Illinois, U.S.A.

This book is protected by copyright. No part of it may be reproduced in any manner without written permission from the publisher.

© 1949 and 1963, by CHARLES C THOMAS • PUBLISHER
Library of Congress Catalog Card Number: 62-21323

First Edition, First Printing, 1949
First Edition, Second Printing, 1950
Second Edition, 1963

With THOMAS BOOKS *careful attention is given to all details of manufacturing and design. It is the Publisher's desire to present books that are satisfactory as to their physical qualities and artistic possibilities and appropriate for their particular use.* THOMAS BOOKS *will be true to those laws of quality that assure a good name and good will.*

Printed in the United States of America

To the Memory of

Dr. William Darrach
and
Dr. Clay Ray Murray

FOREWORD

As the author has pointed out, the modern use of scientifically developed and therapeutically prescribed exercise is not a new development in the field of medicine. However, due to the wartime and postwar interest in rehabilitation and physical medicine, it is today receiving more and more attention. This interest has been strengthened by the emphasis which recently has been placed on early ambulation, an increased understanding of the deconditioning phenomena of bed rest and the recognition that harmful psychological sequelae often result from inactivity during extended hospitalization.

Therapeutic exercise is the foundation of rehabilitation since all subsequent rehabilitation processes are built upon the residual physical disability which medical and surgical care cannot eliminnate. The greatest therapeutic tool in physical medicine is the retaining of the physical residuals of the disabled patient to their maximum effectiveness.

In this book on therapeutic exercise, the author has given both the "why" and the "how." Rather than develop a long list of exercises "to be done in the following manner" as is too frequently done in books on exercise, the book is devoted to fundamental knowledge of exercise therapy and the practical application of such knowledge to specific conditions. That the author through his broad experience and his carefully documented observation knows both the "why" and the "how" of therapeutic exercise is shown by this book which represents a significant contribution to a field of therapy which has not in the past been given the attention it merits.

Howard A. Rusk, M.D.
Professor and Chairman
Department of Rehabilitation
and Physical Medicine
New York University
College of Medicine

INTRODUCTION

THE MODERN development of therapeutic exercises goes back to the work of Ling* who founded, in 1813, the Royal Gymnastic Central Institute in Stockholm. Ling's pupils spread his teachings, and one of them, George H. Taylor, was the author of *An Exposition of the Swedish Movement Cure* (1868), the first book on therapeutic exercises to be published in the United States. Interest in the subject grew very slowly at first. In the past few years, however, the value of therapeutic exercise has been definitely accepted.

During this brief period in which exercises have been admitted to the field of therapy, a trend has started toward specialization in various exercise "systems" for special conditions. Thus, there are to be found exercise specialists for posture, for poliomyelitis, for cerebral palsy, for trauma, for breathing, etc.

Specialization within a specialized field such as therapeutic exercises possesses certain merits, but it possesses great drawbacks as well. Adherence to a single system of treatment usually leads to poor results: the patient is fitted into a treatment procedure instead of the procedure's being shaped to meet the patient's needs. Any system is bound to overlook possibilities offered by other systems and is bound to exclude or neglect helpful details or even useful modes of approach to a problem. Frequently these systems have adherents with emotional, almost religious, fervor. Such an emotional attitude necessarily obscures reason and logic and retards the finding and understanding of important facts. The combination of several systems may represent an improvement, but not a solution. Nor does the sum total

---

* Per Hendrik Ling, 1776-1839. As well as being a man of letters, Ling was, from 1805, fencing master at Lund University, where he developed his system of gymnastics described in *The Gymnastic Free Exercises of Per Hendrik Ling* (trans. 1853). (Cf. C. F. Westerblad: *Ling, His Significance and His Work*, 1907.)

of a number of different systems furnish a satisfactory basis for the use of therapeutic exercises.

The most urgent need for newcomers to this field is a rational basis, a *common denominator,* to meet the variety of problems.

The necessity increases to look at therapeutic exercises as *one whole field,* with numerous subdivisions. Special departments and clinics for the treatment of poliomyelitis, cerebral palsy, postural correction, trauma, etc., retain a definite value in the study and progress of therapeutic exercises. The practical application of therapeutic exercises, however, is likely to be more and more in the hands of those who will have to deal with two or more, possibly all, of the various specialities. Most physical therapists, many nurses, and a growing circle of doctors will desire information in this field. Their greatest interest will not be in elaborate treatises on one speciality, but fundamental knowledge of exercise therapy. For instance, when are exercises indicated? On what basis should they be prescribed? What details are important in exercise techniques? These are some of the questions that are being raised.

It is the aim of this book to suggest a basis for rational prescription and application of exercises, and to establish a number of simple rules directly applicable to individual cases. This must of necessity remain an attempt. Since the history of therapeutic exercises is a relatively brief one, the link between exercises and their foundation in physiology and pathology has not been completed. Much exercise therapy still rests, therefore, on an empirical basis.

There are two main divisions of therapeutic exercises: (a) exercises with the aim of affecting *local muscle* development, exercises that attempt to improve muscle action in small or larger regions of the body; and (b) *general exercises*, the aim of which is principally to produce changes; i.e., improvement of metabolism, circulation, *general* muscle power or *general* relaxation. In this division, development of individual muscle groups or body regions is of secondary or no interest. It is mainly with the first group—exercises concerned with localized muscle improvement—that this book deals. This part of therapeutic exercises occupies the foreground of contemporary interest and discussion, and it is here that the gap between therapeutic exercises and their physiology is widest, that common denominators are most urgently needed.

The section on General Exercises (Part III) attempts merely to give an outline of the great potentialities that have barely been touched upon in practical application. General exercises, as a part of rehabilitation, are far from being routine even in large hospitals. Only since the armed services have included general exercises in their rehabilitation program and since advocators like Rusk and Deaver have worked toward it, has the door been opened to this field of therapeutic exercises.

The immediate demand throughout medicine and surgery is still for special, local effects.

Part I of this book, therefore, stresses the problems of local exercises, though, since local and general exercises cannot be completely separated, many of the suggestions made in this section may be applied to general exercises too. The first chapter tries to establish the fundamentals of exercises as based on clinical physiology and pathology. It attempts to describe the basic qualities of muscle function, the way in which these qualities can be changed in pathological conditions and the way they can be improved by exercises. The next chapter outlines a method of testing and measuring such fundamental qualities of muscle function. Chapter 3 outlines the means, that is, the technique, of how to effect these changes. A special chapter (4) is devoted to the management of pain and painful muscle spasm. The two chapters on exercise prescription and additional instructions to the patient should help in establishing an exercise program and in writing exercise prescriptions in departments of physical medicine.

Part II should serve mainly as an example of how to apply the general principles to particular fields. It is by no means intended to cover all, or even a majority of, the various cases requiring therapeutic exercises. Section 1 on exercises for Muscular-Skeletal Conditions offers a sample of treatment for many types of local disabilities, whether produced by injury or by disease. The section on the Nervous System demonstrates the application of general rules to the special requirements of that field. The same is true of the third section on Respiration. Part III (General Exercises), as indicated, is merely a brief outline of this wide field.

The newcomers to the field of therapeutic exercises for whom this book is intended should possess sufficient background of physiology, pathology, anatomy and kinesiology, so that details have been omitted as far as possible.

Study of the normal is the basis for study of the abnormal and pathological in medicine. This principle should be extended to therapeutic exercises. It is the writer's hope that theoretical and practical study of exercises for the normal may become a large part of the training of every person giving therapeutic exercises. The author has spent many years in theoretical and practical study and teaching of physical exercise and considers it an extremely valuable background. Furthermore, he has endeavored to remain constantly in touch with active treatment of the patient, that is, with the actual giving of exercise treatment; and he feels that this aspect should be much more emphasized in the curricula of doctors interested in therapeutic exercises.

The giving of therapeutic exercises is a craft. As such, it can only be perfected by doing, not by theoretical study. This book can, therefore, serve as a guide but never as a substitute for the actual practice of therapeutic exercises.

Illustrations of the exercises attempted to indicate *"quality"* of muscle function as well as the movement performed (see Figs. 31 and 32). Therefore, the commonly used "stick men" have been abandoned and line drawings have been used. The muscles to which the exercise is directed are marked *black* when the purpose of the exercise is to increase power and *white* when the purpose is to increase elasticity. This way of illustrating the exercises is followed as consistently as possible. It is used when illustrating muscle tests and omitted only when it interferes with clarity of the drawing.

New York City   H.K.

ACKNOWLEDGMENTS
TO FIRST EDITION

THE PUBLICATION of this book has been made possible through the direct and indirect help of a great number of people. I wish to express my most sincere thanks to all of them, although their number preclude my mentioning more than a limited few.

My primary indebtedness is to my teachers:

Dr. William Darrach and Dr. Clay R. Murray, to whom this book is dedicated and whose names will always be remembered with respect by all who believe in a functional approach to traumatic and orthopedic surgery;

Dr. W. Denk, in whose hospital at the University of Vienna I received my early training in fracture surgery and under whose auspices I had the opportunity to organize my first clinics for therapeutic exercises;

Mr. H. Kowalski, to whom I owe much of my knowledge of normal exercises and some invaluable fundamentals for therapeutic exercises, as well as the incentive to study physical education. Mr. Kowalski's ideas regarding the immediate mobilization of strains and sprains inspired my first use of surface anesthesia in the treatment of these injuries; and,

Dr. Harold A. Bruce, the great coach and athlete, who added immeasurably to my training in this field.

Many patients and the constant cooperation of first class treatment teams are required to provide the clinical experience without which a book of this kind is worthless. For their unceasing interest and help I am deeply grateful to many of the Departments of the Columbia Presbyterian Medical Center; particularly Dr. Rustin McIntosh, head of Babies Hospital and his staff, Dr. Harrison McLaughlin, chief of the Fracture Service and his staff, Dr. Frank Stinchfield, Medical Director of the Institute for the Crippled and Disabled; the staff of the Department of Medicine and Dr. Barbara Stimson, who organized and directed the "Low Back Clinic," as well as her successor as chief of this clinic, Dr. Sawnie G. Gaston.

More recently, Dr. Howard A. Rusk has afforded me an unparalleled opportunity to increase my experience in both teaching and clinical work. His associates, Dr. George G. Deaver and Dr. Donald A. Covalt, also have materially contributed to the progress and development of my work.

Among my many co-workers in the field of therapeutic exercises. I am particularly indebted to Mrs. Sonia Weber, whose influence on my thinking and practical exercise work has been considerable. Mrs. Weber's posture work and her work with children have been of great value and have materially contributed to the shaping of the profession. I also wish to thank: Mrs. Edith Hansen, Chief Therapist at Columbia Medical Center and her staff; the staff of the Institute of Rehabilitation and Physical Medicine at New York University; and, my own office therapists, Miss Donna Sheiman and Miss Phyllis Tracy.

For their patient review and constructive criticism of the manuscript, I wish to express my appreciation to Dr. James Blunt of Columbia Medical Center, Miss Elisabeth Addoms, Director of the School of Physical Therapy of New York University, Miss Floy Pinkerton, Associate Director of Training Courses for Physical Therapists at Columbia University and Miss Mary Stuart, Supervisor of the Association for the Aid of Crippled Children.

I am obliged to Mr. Franz Hoellering, the well-known author, for his valuable suggestions regarding the editing and final arrangement of the book and to Miss Jane Meuer and Miss Isabel Athey for their careful work in the preparation of the actual manuscript.

H. K.

CONTENTS

	Page
Foreword	vii
Introduction	ix
Acknowledgments to First Edition	xiii

PART 1
FUNDAMENTAL WORKING PRINCIPLES

Chapter

1. CLINICAL PATHO-PHYSIOLOGY OF MUSCLE EXERCISES 5
    - Muscle Strength 8
        1. Physiology of Muscle Strength 8
        2. Pathology of Muscle Strength 12
        3. Development of Muscle Strength 13
    - Total Elasticity 18
        1. Physiology of Total Elasticity 18
        2. Pathology of Total Elasticity 20
    - Coordination 24
        1. Physiology of Coordination 24
        2. Pathology of Coordination 26
        3. Development of Coordination 26
    - Recommended Reading 27
2. MEASUREMENTS 29
    - The "Motor-Chain" 29
    - Requirements of Muscle Testing 30
    - Measurement of Muscle Strength 31
    - Measurement of Muscle Elasticity 33
    - Measurement of Coordination 36
    - Recording Measurements 38
    - Recommended Reading 39
3. EXERCISE TECHNIQUES 40

Chapter	Page
Exercise Treatment and the Teaching of Exercises	40
Building the Exercise Period	44
Exercise Technique	45
Strength-Building Exercises	45
Elasticity-Developing Exercises	48
Coordination Exercises	51
Group Work	53
Exercise Apparatus	53
Recommended Reading	54
4. TREATMENT OF PAIN AND PAINFUL MUSCLE SPASM	55
Definition	55
Common Treatment Principles	61
The Use of Heat	61
The Use of Surface Anesthetics	62
Evaluation of Pain in the Case History	67
Recommended Reading	68
5. THE EXERCISE PRESCRIPTION	69
Body Region To Be Exercised	69
Exact Type and Form of Exercises	71
Prescription of Dosage	73
6. SUPPORTIVE PRESCRIPTION (and Other Additions to the Treatment)	77
Clothing Habits	77
Working Hazards	81
Childhood Patterns	83
Athletic Activities	83
The Patient's Attitude	86

PART 2

THE APPLICATION OF THERAPEUTIC EXERCISES TO PARTICULAR FIELDS

7. MUSCULO-SKELETAL APPARATUS	91
Indications for Therapeutic Exercises	91
Contra-Indications	98

Chapter	Page
Back	99
Posture	100
Structural Measurements	101
Functional Measurements	103
Muscle Strength and Holding Power Measurements	104
Interpretation of Measurements	107
Interpretation of Structural Measurements	107
Interpretation of Functional Measurements	108
Muscle Length and Elasticity	108
Muscle Strength and Holding Power	108
Posture Exercises	109
Breathing Exercises	109
Stretch of Gastrocnemius Soleus	110
Abdominal Exercises	110
Exercises for Upper Trunk and Shoulder Girdle	113
Exercises for Back Mobility and Rotation	114
Exercises for Hamstring Stretch and Back Mobility	115
Neck Exercises	116
Unilateral Exercises	117
Scoliosis Exercises	118
Foot Exercises	122
Back Pain	124
Strengthening Exercises for Abdominal Muscles (Graded)	127
Strengthening for Hip Flexors	128
Strengthening for Back Muscles	128
Stretching for Hamstring and Back Muscles	129
Acute Back Pain	132
The Neck	135
Acute	135
Chronic	136
Congenital Torticollis (Wry Neck)	136
The Upper Extremity	137
Acute Injury to the Shoulder Girdle	138
Fracture of the Clavicle	138

Chapter	Page
Fracture of the Head of the Humerus	140
Achromio-Clavicular Dislocation	142
Dislocation of the Shoulder Joint	142
Acute Bursitis of the Shoulder	143
Chronic Bursitis of the Shoulder	145
Acute Injury to the Muscles of the Shoulder	146
Fracture of the Shaft of the Humerus	146
Fracture of the Distal End of the Humerus and Intra-Articular Fractures of the Elbow Joint	146
Elbow Joint Dislocations	147
Chronic Injury to the Elbow Region (Tennis Elbow)	147
Fracture of the Forearm	148
Fracture of Distal End of Radius (Colles Fracture)	149
Injury to Small Bones of the Wrist	150
Chronic Conditions of the Wrist Joint	150
Fracture of Metacarpal Bones	151
Fracture of the Fingers	151
The Lower Extremities	152
The Hip Joint (Fracture of the Neck of the Femur)	153
Osteoarthritis of Hipjoint	155
Congenital Dislocations of the Hip	156
Acute Injuries to the Muscles of the Hip and Thigh	157
Chronic Strains of Hip and Thigh Muscles	159
Fracture of the Shaft of the Femur	159
Knee (Fracture of the Patella)	161
Intra-Articular Injuries of the Knee Joint	162
Sprain, Partial Tear of Ligamentous Apparatus of the Knee Joint	163
Chronic Conditions of the Knee Joint	166
Fracture of the Condyles of the Tibia	168
Fracture of the Shaft of the Tibia and Fibula	168
The Ankle and Foot (Fracture of the Ankle)	170
Sprain of the Ankle Joint	170
Fracture of the Short Bones of the Foot	173

Chapter	Page
Chronic Complaints	173
Recommended Reading	176
8. THE NERVOUS SYSTEM	179
General Indications and Technique for Therapeutic Exercises	179
Lower Motor Neuron Lesion	181
General Aspects	181
Peripheral Nerves	183
Injury to the Axillary Nerve	183
Radical Nerve Paralysis	184
Bell's Palsy	185
Lesions to Peripheral Nerve of the Lower Extremity	186
Plexus Injuries	188
Muscle Dystrophies	189
Lesions of the Spinal Cord (Poliomyelitis)	191
Transsection of Spinal Cord	197
Paraplegia	198
Multiple Sclerosis	199
Tabes Dorsalis	200
Lesions to Upper Motor Neuron and Upper Motor Centers	201
Congenital Lesions of Upper Motor Neuron and Upper Motor Centers	201
Cerebral Palsies	201
Types of Exercises Prescribed	208
Rigidity	212
Motor Retardations	212
Post-Natal and Adult Lesions to the Upper Motor Neuron	213
Spastic Hemiplegia	214
Example of a Spastic Hemiplegia	215
Exercise Program	215
Adult Ataxias	216
Recommended Reading	216
9. RESPIRATION	218
Indications	218
Formative Influence on the Chest	219

Chapter	Page
Technique	220
Breathing Muscles Proper (Chest, Intercostals, Diaphragm)	220
Exercises for Auxiliary Breathing Muscles	222
Scaleni, Pectorals, Anterior Serratus, Abdominals	222
Breathing Exercises as Part of Other Exercise Programs (Posture Exercises)	222
Cerebral Palsy	225
Special Pulmonary Conditions (Asthma)	225
In Emphysema	227
After Operation	227
Recommended Reading	228

PART 3
GENERAL EXERCISES

10. GENERAL EXERCISES	231
Indications, Dosage	231
Convalescent Exercises	233
Exercises for Nervous Tension	236
Preventive Exercises	239
Recommended Reading	239
Index	241

THERAPEUTIC EXERCISE

PART 1
FUNDAMENTAL WORKING PRINCIPLES

Chapter 1

CLINICAL PATHO-PHYSIOLOGY OF MUSCLE EXERCISES

PREPARING AND carrying out a therapeutic exercise program on a basis of rational planning and not chance means to *DIRECT* the *proper type* and *amount* of exercise to *the muscles* requiring treatment. It is necessary to know *what* body region or muscle groups we wish to affect and *how* we wish to affect them. We have, therefore to decide, first, what muscle groups are involved (i.e., require exercise) and, secondly, in what *way* we hope to change these muscles.

It is hard to find full explanations and guidance for the physiology of local muscle reactions to exercises. The facts directly applicable to therapeutic exercise work are scattered and it therefore seems advisable to give a brief outline of applied *physiology* and pathology as regards the *local effect of exercise**. . . . .

For *clinical purposes we may differentiate three basic qualities of muscle function:*

1. The ability of a muscle to contract—*strength*.
2. The ability of a muscle to give up contraction and to yield to passive stretch: total—*elasticity*.
3. The ability of a muscle to co-operate with other muscles in

---

* A knowledge of body mechanics is the first requirement and can be acquired from any of the numerous reliable books on muscle anatomy and *kinesiology*. A knowledge of muscle *physiology*, the second requirement, cannot, however, be so readily derived from these textbooks for the purpose of understanding normal and pathological muscle function. A considerable part of the material in these books deals with physiological effects on respiration, metabolism and circulation. These effects of exercise on the organism are important when therapeutic exercises are given with the intention of affecting the whole body. This part of muscle physiology will not be described here except for references, in connection with special problems, in the chapters on *General Exercises in Convalescence,* and *Exercises in Cardiac Cases.*

proper timing and with appropriate power and elasticity—*co-ordination.*

The purpose of therapeutic exercises is—to improve—one or more of these qualities. This is done by calling upon (exercising) the quality sought.

A muscle quality used often enough and intensely enough will increase.

If a muscle function is not repeated frequently enough in any single exercise period, or if a sufficient number of periods per week is not maintained, or not carried on for the necessary number of weeks, no increase of the quality sought can be expected.

If the movements performed are not identical, different muscles and different qualities will be used in a different way each time. Thus repetition (identical function of the same muscles) will not occur and the muscle quality will not be developed as desired.

Muscle Function

Qualities	Pathology	Therapeutic Exercises
Strength (Contraction)	Weakness	Strengthening Exercises (Resistance, weight)
Total Elasticity		
Physiological Elasticity (Relaxation)	Tension	Relaxing Exercises
	Spasm	Relaxing Exercises and Relief of Pain
	Spasticity	Relaxing Exercises
	Rigidity	Relaxing Exercises
Mechanical Elasticity (Yielding to Passive stretch)	Contracture	Stretching Exercises, Active and Passive
Coordination	Incoordination	Strengthening, Relaxing Stretching if Needed Then Coordination (Accomplishment) Exercises

Fig. 1

If the function desired is not performed with enough *intensity* (in high enough dosage) to exceed the present demand for it, no increase of that quality can be expected.

Repeated performance of a function in large enough dosage will cause the development of the quality called for.

Identical functions of muscles can be produced only if identical movements are carried out. This prerequisite is obtained solely by keeping all elements involved in the motion the same. These elements are:
1. The muscles involved.
2. The qualities sought in these muscles.
3. The speed of performance.
4. The rest-period between performances.
5. The range of movement caused by the performance.
6. The intensity of effort involved.

The sum-total of all these elements of a movement constitute the *form* of the movement.

A movement prescribed and performed in proper form, and aimed at the development of a given muscle quality or qualities, is a *therapeutic exercise*.

If an exercise is repeated frequently enough in the same form and in sufficient and correct dosage, it will develop the *quality sought*. This value of an exercise—the ability of an exercise to develop a given quality—we call *exercise value*.

As mentioned before, three basic muscle qualities are of main interest:

(1) **Muscle contraction*** the normal reaction of a muscle to stimuli, which is the source of *Muscle Strength;*

(2) **Total elasticity**, the ability of a muscle to give up contraction and assume a maximum length; and,

(3) **Co-ordination**, the properly timed and adequate response of a muscle by contraction and elasticity in co-operation with the other muscles or muscle groups. A muscle in the body does not act by itself, but in combination with many other muscles.

It is possible in most cases to explain a deficiency in muscle action as the consequence of one, two or all three of these basic qualities. While the pathology, the primary lesion, may have a different seat in every case concerned, the aim common to the treatment of all such conditions will be restoration or improve-

---

* The term, "contraction" is a misnomer; it implies etymologically "shortening." It is used here, in accordance with established practice, as a synonym for *tension*.

ment of the impaired quality. In a weak muscle we should try for strength. In an inelastic muscle we should try for increased elasticity. In a muscle that has lost its *properly timed and correct co-operation* with others, the goal will be to restore proper co-ordination.

As previously stated, a muscle will develop the quality is it called upon to perform. Once we know *what* muscle is deficient (kinesiology) and once we know what quality is deficient, we have only to direct proper exercises to the muscle, *i.e.*, to work toward its improvement. The proper exercises will be those that necessitate the use of the lacking quality, in the proper manner and amount. If we understand these qualities and know how to ask for them, we may obtain them. It will, therefore, be worthwhile to discuss these three basic clinical qualities of skeletal muscle, the conditions under which they are impaired and the type of muscle action that requires, and consequently develops, these qualities.

MUSCLE STRENGTH

1. Physiology of Muscle Strength

Muscle strength is the ability of a muscle to overcome gravity or resistance, and therefore means the ability of the muscle to produce work. The physiological process by which the muscle produces power is called contraction.

A muscle reacts with contraction to stimuli coming normally over the lower motor neuron.

The main criterion of muscle contraction is its increasing tension. This increase of muscle tension can be associated with various phases of muscle length, differentiated as follows (*see* Fig. 2):

(*a*) *Isometric Contraction,* in which the length of the muscle remains the same. This type of contraction produces no movements. The augmented tension of the contracting muscle is matched either by an opposing weight too heavy to allow this increase of tension to result in shortening, or by an equally intense contraction by its antagonist. This isometric muscle contraction does not result in movement but is effective as *holding power.*

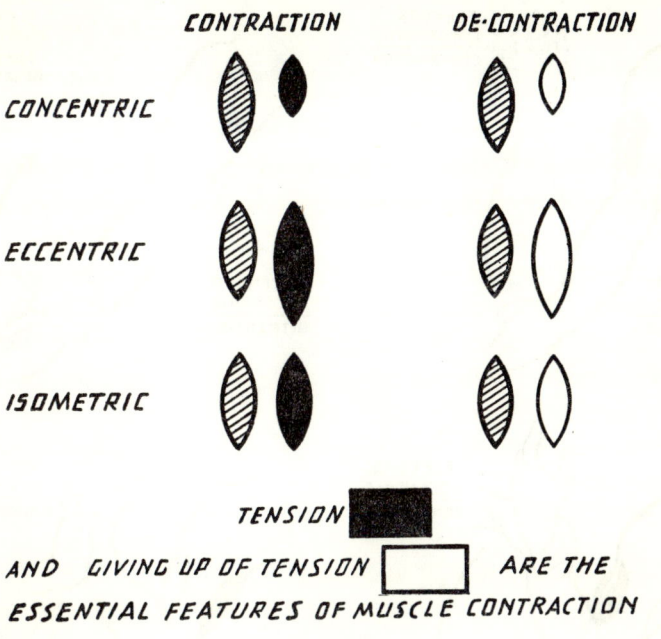

Fig. 2

(b) **Concentric Contraction,** which involves shortening of the muscle. The tension of the muscle may either increase or remain the same. The result of this kind of muscle contraction is movement, with the speed of the movement proportionate to the speed of the shortening of the muscle. The strength with which the movement is executed is proportionate to the increase of tension. This form of power is called moving power, and it ranges from slow motion to fast power movements.

(c) **In Eccentric Contraction** the length of the muscle increases while its tension may remain the same or even increase. This occurs if weight, or resistance, lengthens a muscle but is opposed by persistent or increasing muscle tension.

The ability of a muscle to produce strength—that is, work—

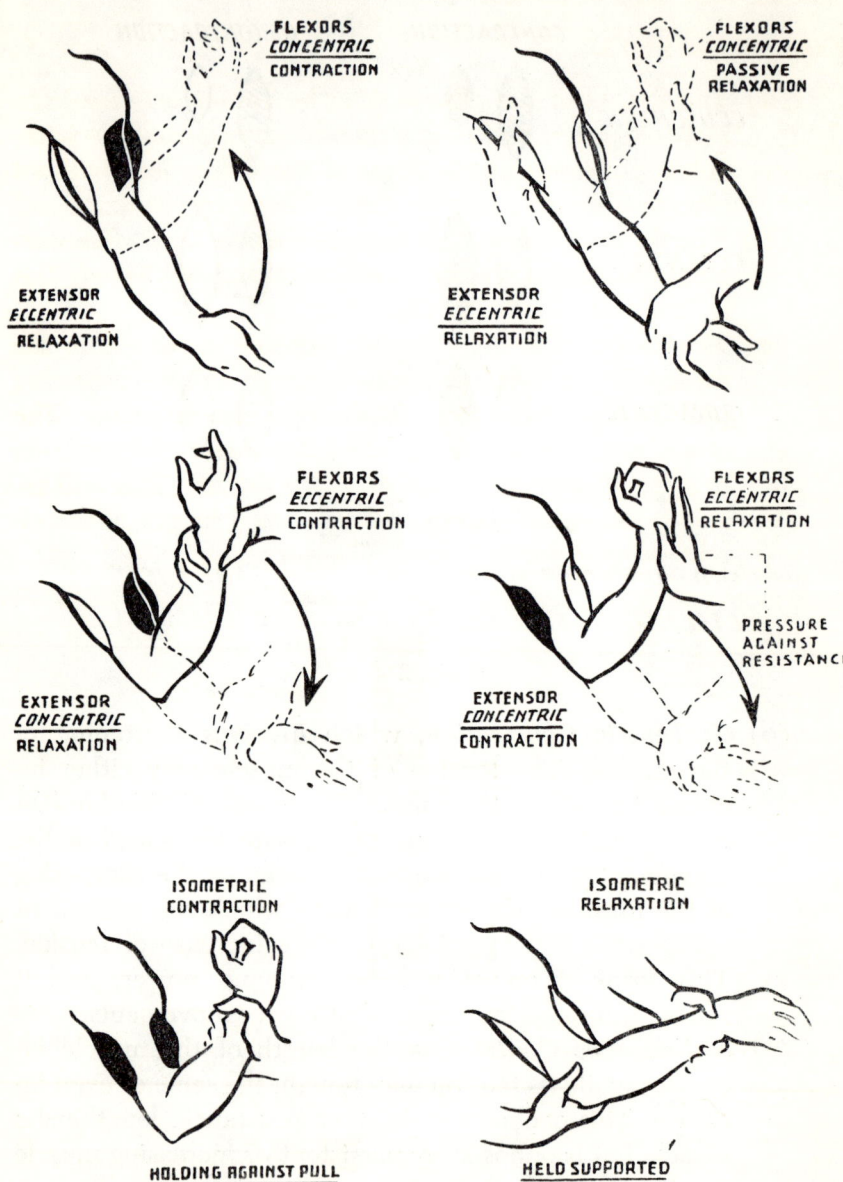

Fig. 3

for a period of time is called *endurance.* Endurance is accounted great if a muscle is able to produce heavy work for extended periods, with little or no rest.

Example *(see* Fig. 3)

(a) The flexors of the elbows may be consciously made to increase in tension, as in a muscle setting exercise, without any movement resulting at the elbow and without change in muscle length: this is "isometric contraction."

(b) The flexors of the elbow may increase in tension and decrease in length when the elbow is actively flexed: this is "concentric contraction."

(c) The flexors of the elbow may increase in tension to the maximum of their capacity against an overpowering pull by an outside force in the opposite direction. The elbow will be forced from a flexed to a stretched position in spite of increased tension in the flexors. This will result in increased tension and increased length in the elbow flexors; this is "eccentric contraction."

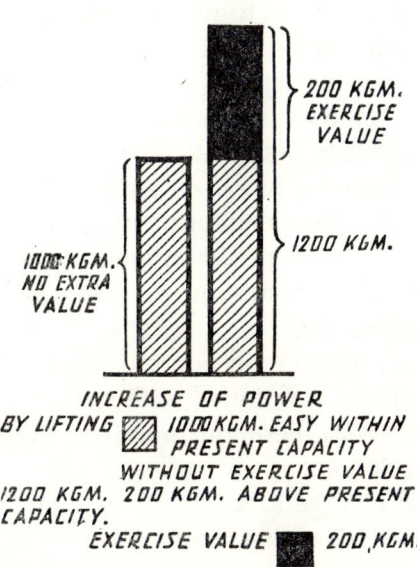

Fig. 4

2. Pathology of Muscle Strength

Muscle strength in all phases can be reduced or lost by inactivity. This inactivity may be imposed (splints, bandages, bed rest) or it may be involuntarily caused by the substitution of a better-fitted muscle for the inactivated one. Consistent lack of use as, for instance, constant sedentary living, may cause relative weakness, in otherwise "normal" individuals.

Substitution takes place if the muscle is weaker than its synergists, if it hurts, if it is contractured or if it does not respond to or does not receive normal nervous stimuli.

Normal, everyday activities, which keep *other synergists* of this muscle strong and active, will not stimulate this particular muscle; it will therefore lag more behind its synergists.

Constant *overstretching* of muscles, making their normal contraction impossible, will cause these muscles to lose power, to weaken. This overstretching may be caused by constant pull, such as that produced by spasm or spasticity of the antagonists, preponderance of antagonists, gravity or other mechanical force. (Supporting splints and avoidance of overtraction are the remedies.)

The ability of a muscle to produce strength can be diminished or completely destroyed by *lesions* of the mucle proper (such as injury or muscle dystrophy) or by lesions of its innervation (lower and upper motor neuron and afferent nerves).

Flaccid paralysis is present if the ability of a muscle to contract upon nerve impulse has been entirely lost. It this paralysis is due to lesion of the lower motor neuron, the muscle proper may possibly still respond to direct stimuli (electrical stimulation, etc.). If, however, the condition persists too long, contractility may be lost permanently.

Lesion of the upper motor neuron may result in flaccid paralysis of certain muscles, combined with spastic paralysis of others. They are called zero cerebral muscles. They may respond to stimuli *via* peripheral nerve reflexes.

The physical change in a muscle that commonly takes place in weakened muscles is called atrophy. If muscle tissue is replaced and apparently increased by non-functional tissue, such as fat, it is called pseudo-hypertrophy.

The effectiveness of muscle contraction may be further reduced by diminished speed or endurance, or by both. The endurance factor is sometimes greatly diminished, with the muscle being unable to perform more than one brief contraction at a time, and requiring a long rest period to make another contraction possible.

3. Development of Muscle Strength (*see* Fig. 4)

Exercises to develop muscle strength call for muscle power —i.e., contraction. Specifically, these exercises have in common the lifting of a weight or the overcoming of resistance. Depending on the other elements of form present in the strength building exercise, different types and variations may be developed:

(a) *Fast moving strength*—by exercises requiring fast contraction: fast movements.
(b) *Slow moving strength*—by exercises requiring slow contraction: slow movements.
(c) *Holding strength*—by exercises without motion other than tensing or by exercises requiring a preponderance of tensing, such as most eccentric contraction.

Strength-building exercises repeated in succession for long periods will develop endurance.

The dosage of strength-building exercises will depend on:

(a) **Amount of contraction** performed *(resistance or gravity given).*
(b) **Number of contractions** performed, and number of performance periods per day, repetition of contractions in the time unit.

Here the question arises as to how much work (resistance—gravity) a muscle has to perform in order to increase its strength as quickly as possible. Should a muscle be worked to fatigue or to well below fatigue limit? This question is partly answered by experience, partly by classical experiment—the Fatigue-Training Graph.

Strength building exercises with too little exercise value do not increase strength or do so only very slowly (Fig. 4). It is essential to give sufficient quantity of strength building work. On the other hand, strength-building exercises given in too large

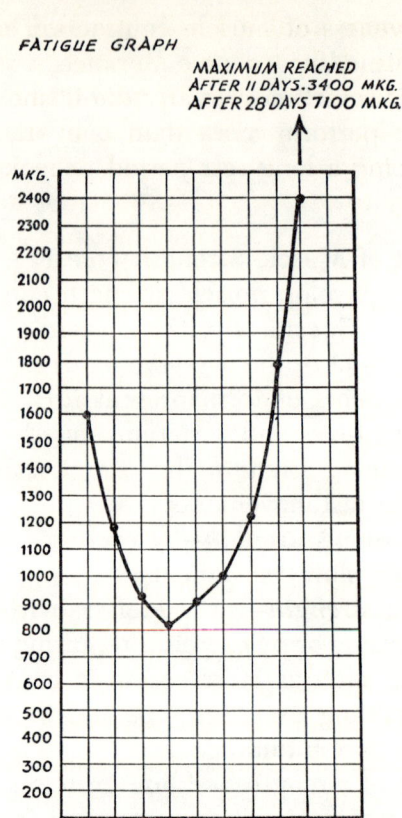

Fig. 5

doses result in pain and decrease of strength, at least temporarily.

The experiment to determine the graph of muscle training was made by recording the maximum weight-lifting capacity of normal persons on consecutive days. It was found (*see* Fig. 5) that the maximum weight that could be lifted was less on the second and fourth days of the experiment. The fifth and sixth days brought a gradual increase in capacity. It took the subjects approximately seven days to regain the weight-lifting capacity of the first day.

From the end of the first week, a continuous gain over the initial capacity could be observed. After the first gains, the graph rose more and more until it finally reached maximum capacity. Discontinuing the daily training resulted in a prompt set-back, which could be prevented only by two training periods a week.

Strength-building exercises should, in the majority of cases, be given *below fatigue.* In very weak muscles fatigue may decrease the ability to exercise so far that the muscles cannot perform at all. Several days of rest may be necessary before resuming exercises. By then the initial gains may have disappeared, and training will have to start all over again—only to produce the same negative results if pushed past the fatigue limit.

Fatigue may increase contractures, produce pain and painful muscle spasm (*see Elasticity,* p. 22). This is one more reason for avoiding fatigue.

The closer the muscles come to normal, the closer will strength-building exercises approach the fatigue limit—or actually reach it.

If the fatigue graph is disregarded, the patient should be informed of the probable consequences. He should be warned of decreasing efficiency, possibly pain, discomfort when his performance follows the downgrade of the graph.

Fatigue limits differ for different types of strength-building exercises, according to different people and to the condition of the muscles in question. In a later discussion of measurements we shall deal with the gauging of muscle strength and the establishment of fatigue limits.

The quality of resistance (or amount of weight) given to the muscle will have a bearing on the strength-building process as well as the number of repetitions.

If taxed with the maximum weight (to the point of real fatigue), a muscle will not immediately be able to perform again, and strength-building work on this level, therefore, will not be possible. If practiced with a minimum weight, frequent repetition is possible, but that does not have sufficient strength-building value because less, not more, strength is being asked for the muscle than it exerts in everyday performance.

The weight (or resistance) given for strength-building purposes must be large enough to demand more than the normal effort of the involved muscle but less than the maximal effort.

Endurance can be developed by emphasizing repetition instead of resistance, but it must be noted that endurance is a function of *strength plus repeated* performance. Endurance for high-powered performance will not be produced by repetition alone: we shall have to build up, at the same time, to heavy resistance and frequent performance to obtain such a result.

In pathology of the muscle, the fatigue limit may be especially low. The same is true of the muscles in which the lower motor neuron has been affected or destroyed. Muscles that have atrophied after local injury, due to non-use, etc., usually are *less sensitive to fatigue* than muscles atrophied as a result of motor nerve lesion. Zero cerebral muscles affected in the upper neuron, or by cerebral injuries, may respond well to sub-cortical stimuli with strong contraction. They can be kept strong or be strengthened by means of confusion. Confusion movements—as yet unexplained—are responses of zero cerebral muscles to certain move-

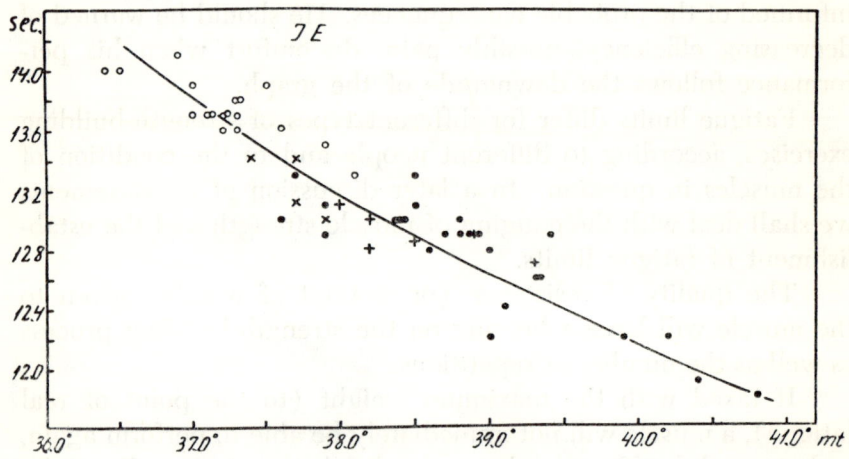

PERFORMANCE TIME FOR SPRINT (956 MKG). PLOTTED AGAINST TEMPERATURE OF LATERAL VASTUS MUSCLE.

O NO "WARMING UP"
● "WARMING UP" BY PRELIMINARY WORK.
+ "WARMING UP" BY DIATHERMY
× WARMING UP BY HOT SHOWER.

COURTESY OF ACTA PHYSIOLOGIA SKANDINAV VOL.10 FASG.1 AUG.2 1945
ERLING ASSMUSSEN & OVE BØJE.

Fig. 6

ments: for example, the reaction of a zero cerebral anterior tibial muscle with dorsi-flexion of the ankle when giving resistance to hip flexion (*see* Figs. 82 and 83).

A similar effect can sometimes be produced by pain-reflex. For example: flexion of knee and hip joints may be caused by forced, painful, passive flexion of the big toe.

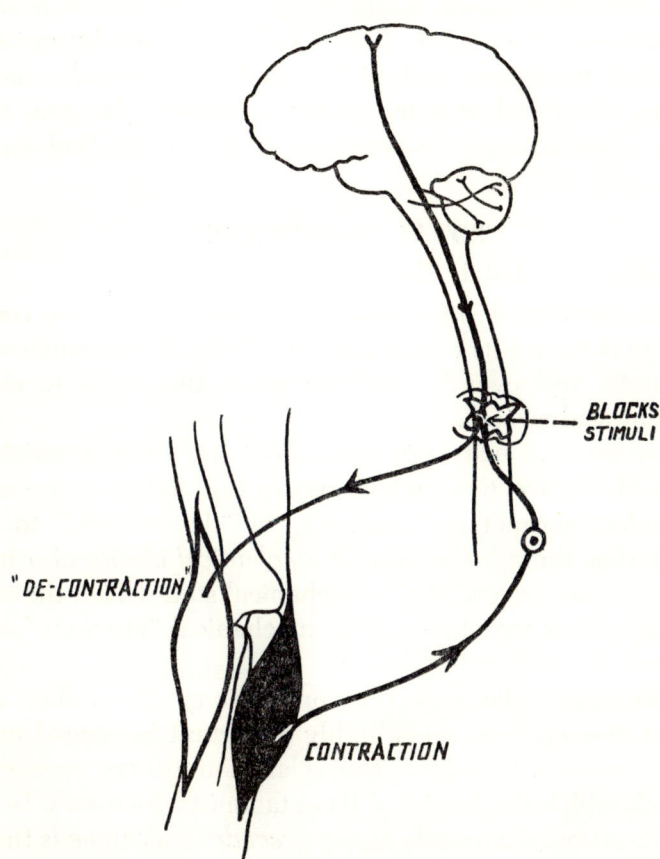

Fig. 7

Holding power can be developed by isometric contraction. This contraction may be brought about by simply holding a position against resistance or by the "tensing" of a muscle. The same result can be obtained by "eccentric" contractions, if "tensing" is emphasized rather than movement.

When giving strength-building exercises—as well as exercises to increase elasticity and co-ordination—the fact of "warm-up" (Fig. 6) has to be considered. A muscle does not function with maximal efficiency unless warmed up by work or—to a slightly lesser extent—by deep heat. This has been shown by measuring the muscle temperature and, at the same time, muscle efficiency in a series of normal persons. (Attention should be paid to this warm-up when arranging an exercise program—*see Technique,* p. 40.)

TOTAL ELASTICITY

1. Physiology of Total Elasticity

Total elasticity is the ability of a muscle to give up contraction and to decrease its tension, thus enabling it to assume a maximum length, and, even beyond this point, the ability to yield to passive physical stretch.

There are *two phases* of total elasticity: First, *physiological elasticity (de-contraction),* which means the ability of the muscle to surrender contraction (tension), to "de-contract," to relax. Added to this, there is the normal *mechanical ability* of a muscle to yield to passive stretching, a mechanical state which the muscle shares with other structures. This mechanical "elasticity" is similar to that of a coil spring.

Physiological elasticity (de-contraction)—the ability of the muscle to give up tension—is highly important in normal motion.

The speed with which the relaxation occurs exceeds the speed with which the length of its antagonists decreases. In other words, relaxation of a muscle group *precedes and exceeds* the contraction of the antagonist, in normal movements. It is the prior relaxation and lengthening of muscles which provides for a smooth movement. The pull by antagonists is not present in normal muscle action. If the elasticity of a muscle is slowed up to such a point that it is unable to precede contraction of its antagonist, the muscle is in danger of being pulled, i.e., injured, by fast antagonist contraction.

Physiological elasticity is an active spontaneous response of a muscle, not a rubber-band stretch produced by the action of its antagonist. As an example: visualize, in slow motion, pictures of runners, the lengthening muscles as they are seen fluttering, relaxed before their length is consumed by completion of the joint movements. The physiological basis for this relaxation preceding contraction of the antagonist is found in experiments that show that, if the flexors of a joint are stimulated, the extensors of this same joint react with relaxation.

A tired muscle loses some of its ability to relax. The endurance of a muscle is therefore characterized not only by its ability to produce power over a prolonged period of time, but also by its ability at the same time to maintain elasticity. *An endurant muscle readily assumes its maximum length after repeated or long contractions.* A fatigued muscle loses part of its ability to return to its maximum length.

Physiological elasticity—the giving up of contraction—relaxation—may be observed in three types, depending on the relation between the length and tenseness of a muscle. *These three types form counterparts of the three types of muscle contraction described under muscle power* (see Fig. 2):

    (a) Isometric relaxation, in which the release of tenseness is not followed by increase in length. No movement results, but the tenseness of the muscle is decreased.

    (b) Eccentric relaxation, in which release of tenseness is combined with increase in length, the common procedure in normal active movement.

    (c) Concentric relaxation, in which decrease of tenseness is associated with decrease of length, a condition present in a relaxed passive movement in which insertion and attachment of the muscle are approximated.

Example (*see* Fig. 3)

    (a) The flexors of the elbow may be fully consciously relaxed without any movement at the elbow joint and without change in muscle length. This is "isometric decontraction" (isometric relaxation).

(b) The flexors of the elbow may be relaxed (decontracted) and lengthened when the elbow is being stretched from a flexed position to full extension. This is "eccentric decontraction" (eccentric relaxation).

(c) The flexors of the elbow may be fully consciously relaxed or decontracted while the elbow is passively carried from a position of extension.

2. Pathology of Total Elasticity

Elasticity in all phases can be diminished by faulty management (either exercising or resting) of a muscle. A muscle kept in a shortened position for a long period of time (or fatigued), will permanently assume the reduced length; the result will be: *contracture*. If a muscle is worked beyond pain limit, it will react with muscle *spasm*.

If in the course of an exercise a muscle is not given time (rest period) or opportunity (return to full length and relaxation) to resume its maximum elasticity, a tendency to residual tension and shortening will develop, leading to loss of elasticity.

If a muscle contracts frequently, in succession, a tendency to maintain contraction develops, and loss of elasticity results—this is especially likely in fatigue.

A weak atrophic muscle is easily fatigued, and is exposed to loss of elasticity sooner than a normal muscle. This is a further reason for keeping exercises below fatigue limit (*see Fatigue Graph*, Fig. 5).

The elasticity of a muscle can be diminished or impaired in:

I. *Impaired Physiological Elasticity:*

(a) **Muscle spasm** is present if the muscle is pathologically forced to maintain a state of tension and shortness (contraction) by stimuli to the lower motor neuron. The most common "painful, peripheral muscle spasm" is due to pain stimuli to the lower motor neuron, causing painful muscle contraction (*see* Fig. 22). This contraction cannot be released like normal contraction, but remains permanent as long as the stimuli subsist and as long as there prevails a vicious circle of pain—contraction—pain. The characteristics of this spasm are pain and disability of a muscle to de-contract.

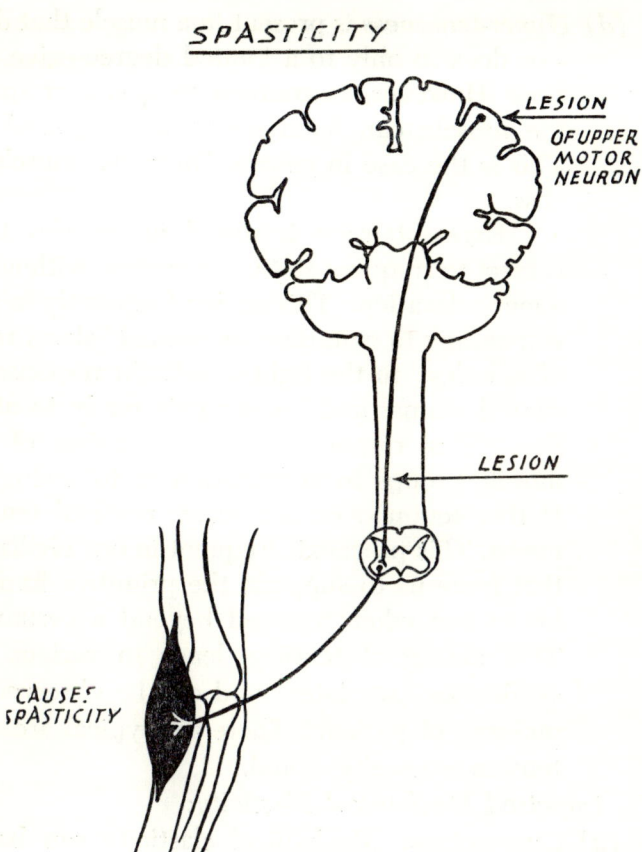

Fig. 8

(b) **Spasticity**: a condition caused by lesion of the upper motor neuron (Fig. 8). In spasticity the muscle reacts with contraction to all stimuli reaching it *via* the central nervous system. It does not de-contract when its antagonists contract, but responds with contraction to the stimulus elicited by the contraction of its antagonists.

*(c) **Rigidity*** is present in a muscle when it only slowly changes (increases) its length, approaching the "pull-by-antagonist" pattern, which normally does not exist.

*(d) **Hyper-tenseness*** is present in a muscle that does not —or does so only to a limited degree—give up tension. However, in contrast to spasm or spasticity, the muscle can lengthen to the required extent. This is the case in general "nervous" muscle tenseness.

Excess tension is stored in muscles that are subject to frequent static contraction without subsequent relaxation. This occurs frequently in persons responding to irritations by normal "alarm reaction" of muscles. In the fight and flight response the irritated animal and human gets ready to attack or flee. This response includes tensing of certain muscle groups in anticipation of following action. If this action does not occur, residual tension remains. This process is frequent in our civilized lives that force us to suppress the primitive impulses to hit or run when irritated beyond a certain point. This storing of tensions leads to various tension syndromes (see later) and can be observed in the majority of patients. There are typical areas where tension is usually stored.

II. *Impaired Mechanical Elasticity*:
  *(a) **Contracture:*** Mechanical elasticity can be diminished permanently. Such a condition, if sufficiently persistent, can be associated with fibrous changes in the *contractured muscles*.
  *(b) **Overstretched Muscles:*** Muscles in which the normal length is exaggerated.

III. *Development of Total Elasticity:* The method used to develop elasticity will depend on what phase is desired (physiological or physical), and on the cause of the loss of elasticity.

(a) **In painful muscle spasm,** the development of physiological elasticity is based on the relief of pain *(see Management of Pain)*, plus movements calling for relaxation of the muscle. These movements may be (1) isometric contractions of the antagonists (pushing against unyielding resistance to bring about reflex relaxation of the muscles in painful spasm), or (2) slow contraction of the antagonist, causing slow relaxation and lengthening of the affected muscle. The same types of movement may be used when the vicious circle of painful spasm is broken by blocking the motor impulses (curare).

(b) **In spasticity** due to upper motor neuron lesion, relaxation has to be attempted by trying for:
  (1) Conscious suppression of muscle contraction. The patient is first taught the feeling of tensing by contracting or tensing a normal muscle group, then the feeling of relaxation after releasing that contraction. This releasing of tenseness is then taught in relation to the affected spastic muscle groups, a process carried out step by step *(see Technique)*.
  (2) De-concentration. The attention of the patient is directed elsewhere while trying for the relaxed movement *(see Technique)*. Attention is directed to other parts or actions of the body, such as breathing, and away from the tense muscles.

(c) **In tenseness,** general relaxation training should be given and supplemented by teaching of local conscious relaxation and habit forming exercises.

(d) **In rigidity,** relaxation is prescribed.

IV. Lack of Physical Elasticity (contracture) can be overcome only by stretching. We speak of stretching a muscle, if its length is increased by forces other than those inherent in the muscle itself. This stretching can be done by pull by the antagonists (Fig. 18) or, passively, by the person treating the patient. It is well to combine this passive stretch with reflex relaxation, because a "rigid" phase may precede the final lengthening phase of the muscle (*see* Fig. 19).

Never stretch a tensed muscle before relaxing it.

Passive stretch can be performed by weights (traction). The weights used to produce stretching have to be attached by loops or adhesive to the extremity—they cannot be actively held by the patient's hand (*see* Fig. 20).

COORDINATION

1. Physiology of Coordination

Coordination is the well-timed and well-balanced function of several muscles together. It is the well-timed play of proper contraction and de-contraction (relaxation), which produces useful movements, proper body posture and placement of the limbs in space, and proper relation of the various parts of the body to one another.

By means of the central nervous system, the muscles are not only linked with the motor sphere in the brain and thereby enabled to respond to voluntary impulses, but a number of subcortical centers afford connection between all the parts of the body and these muscles. These centers link the function of individual muscles and muscle groups to various incoming stimuli from organs governing equilibrium, vision, state of contraction of other muscles, joints, etc.; the steady flow of impulses provides for certain, though varying, degree of contraction in all normal muscles in a healthy body.

Reflexes are a part of this complicated reaction of muscles to occurrences within and outside the body. Some of these reflexes have been mentioned in connection with strength, others in connection with elasticity. Other reflexes have an important bearing on the understanding of the exercises, such as:

Postural Reflexes: These are of proprioceptive nature, that is, they are reactions to movements by other parts of the body, to positioning of the body, gravity and reaction to external sensory stimuli. Residual tension often influences posture, especially if target area of that tension is in neck or shoulder girdle muscles.

Placing the body in certain positions provokes reflex movements. This is especially true if the influence of the mind — volition — is negligible — for instance in babies. Positioning reflexes can, in these cases, be used as a means of inducing movements desired for their exercise value. For example: placing a baby over the edge of a bed, with its pelvis and legs dangling, will cause pulling up of both legs, flexing of knees, contraction of abdominal muscles (Fig. 16).

Conditioned Reflexes (responses): As an example: the presence of food will evoke the flow of saliva in a dog. If a musical note is sounded each time the food is offered, the sound by itself will—after sufficient repetition of the experiment— provoke salivation.

This method of causing a response to stimuli that normally do not provoke such reactions can be used to elicit muscle action as well as the gland-function in this classical experiment (Pavlov). In this field, conditioned "blinking," "tongue-motions" and other movements have been demonstrated. The ready response of a ball player when catching or hitting the ball at the right moment, the fast counterblow and parrying of a blow by a boxer, are all greatly dependent on conditioned responses.

Conditioning exercises are used, either when voluntary response is not forthcoming (in children), or when a substitution for voluntary action by involuntary action (habit) is desired.

With children the singing of nursery rhymes to the accompaniment of passive motion will "condition" the child to *move spontaneously* upon hearing the tune.

Linking an exercise with a frequently occurring episode of daily life will produce a *habit:* the "conditioned" repetition of this exercise whenever the linked-up episode takes place. For example "to bend and stretch knees when getting up from a chair and when sitting down" will produce the repeated movement and will be of help in cases of "rest pain."

Movements are produced by the concerted action of several muscles, and are made up of contractions of one group and decontractions of others. Changes in muscle length and tenseness occur in varying degrees. The simplest movement, therefore, constitutes a combination of many different muscle actions in several muscles and muscle groups. It constitutes a *movement pattern* rather than an action of a single muscle.

The complex teamwork of numerous muscles, plus the mechanical effort of different leverage, causes different degrees of strength and elasticity to be present at different sectors of a joint range. Every sector of this range will differ from others in maximum muscle strength and in maximum potential elasticity.

2. Pathology of Coordination

In all previously described disturbances of muscle strength (*see* p. 12) and of elasticity (*see* p. 20) or of both, the affected muscle will not be able to co-operate, in a well-timed and well-balanced manner, with its synergists and antagonists. If the disfunction is of minor degree, this disability may be hidden by other, compensating muscles. When disfunction is severe enough, it will be obvious and will result in poor coordination or lack of it (incoordination). This incoordination will be the more obvious, the more complicated the movement patterns.

Poor coordination may be due to incorrect timing and incorrect quantitative cooperation of certain muscles, even though strength and elasticity are perfect. The cause may be lesions of the central nervous system.

If motor patterns cannot be established, or if they have been forgotten, the symptom of "incoordination" may appear. This is true physiologically of learning new skills. A child learning how to walk, a person learning how to ride a bicycle offer good examples of "normal" incoordination.

3. Development of Coordination

Coordination may be developed by developing elasticity or strength if either of these qualities are impaired.

Simple movement patterns should be performed if lack of coordination is due to lesion of the central nervous system. The simple patterns are then made complicated step by step. In balance training, simple balance pictures are developed into more complicated balance performance.

In involuntary motion, lack of coordination is the consequence of inability to suppress movement: irregular movements will result. Repetition of movement patterns is useless, because involuntary movements are irregular. However, involuntary movements can be reduced by learning how to suppress impulses to contract muscles—by learning relaxation. This relaxation can be achieved directly or indirectly, depending on the individual case—rarely by reflex relaxation.

Poor coordination may result from relative over-development of one quality in a muscle, or from poor elasticity or poor power or from both of the last. Attempting skills too far beyond capacity also may aggravate poor coordination. Therefore, in developing coordination, the gradual increase of the task, the step-by-step procedure, is especially important.

RECOMMENDED READING

ALTSCHULE, MARK D.: *Bodily Physiology in Mental and Emotional Disorders.* New York, Grune & Stratton, 1953.

BUCHTHAL, FRITZ AND KAISER, E.: Factors determining tension development in skeletal muscle. *Acta physiol. Scandinav.* 8:38-74, 1944.

CANNON, WALTER B.: *Bodily Changes in Pain, Hunger, Fear and Rage,* 2nd ed. New York, Appleton & Co., 1929.

———————: The mechanism of emotional disturbance of bodily functions. *New England J. Med.,* pp. 887-884, 1928.

DE LORME, THOMAS L., FERRIS, B. J. AND GALLAGHER, ROSWELL J.: Effect of progressive resistance exercise on muscle contraction time. *Arch. Phys. Med.,* XXXIII: No. 2, Feb. 1952.

DUNBAR, H. F.: *Emotions and Bodily Changes.* New York, Columbia University Press, 1935.

ELFTMAN, H.: The action of muscles in the body. *Biol. Symp.,* 3:191-209, 1941.

ERLING, ASMUSSEN: Ove Boje. Body temperature and capacity for work. *Acta physiol. scandinav.,* 10: Fascl., 1945.

FULTON, JOHN F.: *Howell's Textbook of Physiology.* Philadelphia and London, W. E. Saunders Co., 1946.

———————: *Muscular Contraction and the Reflex Control of Movement.* Baltimore, Williams & Wilkins, 1926.

KRAUS, HANS: Clinical pathophysiology of therapeutic exercise. *New York State J. Med.,* p. 294, Feb. 1949.

LIDDELL, E. G., AND SHERRINGTON, CHARLES S.: Reflexes in response to strength (myotatic reflexes). *Proc., Roy. Soc.,* (B.) 96:212-242, 1925.

MACKENZIE, COLLIN: *The Action of Muscles.* New York, Paul B. Hoeber, Inc., 1940.

MAGNUS, R.: Some results of studies in the physiology of posture (Cameron Price Lectures). *Lancet,* 2:531-536, 585-588, 1926.

PAVLOV, I. P.: *Conditioned Reflexes: An Investigation of the Physiological Activities of the Cerebral Cortex.* London, Oxford University Press, 1927.

SAINSBURY, P. AND GIBSON, J. G.: Symptoms of anxiety and tension and the accompanying physiological changes in the muscular system. *J. Neurol.* (British) *17*:216, August 1954.

SELYE, HANS: *The Story of the Adaptation Syndrome.* Med. Publishers, Montreal, Canada, 1962.

SHERRINGTON, CHARLES S.: Reciprocal innervation of antagonistic muscles: 14th note on double reciprocal innervation. *Proc. Roy. Soc.,* (B) *81*: 249-268, 1909.

STEINDLER, ARTHUR: *Mechanics of Normal and Patholigical Locomotion in Man.* Springfield, Thomas, 1935.

TIEGEL, E.: Ueber Muskelkontraktur im Gegensatz zur Kontraktion. *Pfluger's Archives fuer de Ges. Physiol.,* 13:71, 1876.

Chapter 2

MEASUREMENTS

I<small>N THE FOREGOING</small> chapter the basic qualities of muscle physiology that may serve as common denominators for an exercise program have been described. In addition it has been emphasized that prescribing the correct amount—the proper dosage—is just as important as assigning the correct type of exercise. This consideration at once brings up the necessity of measuring the muscle quantity that we have undertaken to improve by exercise.

These measurements and muscle tests serve two purposes: (1) to help establish a basis for the exercise program; and, (2) to help evaluate progress or regression.

Electrical and ergometric tests require special equipment and will not be described here. This discussion will be confined to simple tests needing either no instruments or only primitive measuring devices. The more elaborate tests, which are more exact in degree, and sometimes more informative, are limited to special cases or case groups; it is difficult to use them in daily clinical work because they take too much time.

All these measurements, particularly the simple measurements here described, furnish only relative and approximate figures; this holds true to a lesser degree for the more elaborate ones. While these measurements are important in gauging relative muscle values, they do not represent mathematically exact values.

THE "MOTOR-CHAIN"

When testing a human muscle, it must be remembered that with it the whole "motor-chain" is tested. This chain includes the skeleton and joints, and the central nervous system with peripheal nerves as well as the psychological attitudes and responses of the patient. Testing of this motor-chain must be done under identical conditions if comparable results are to be obtained.

However, such similarity of conditions is nearly impossible. While we may be able to re-establish identical conditions for skeleton and joints, it is impossible to do so for muscles and for the nervous system, because of the various reflexes and, to a much greater extent, the influence of the cortex and subcortical centers. Conditions can be indentical only when denervated muscle is tested in experiments. Normally the element of volition, the element of reflex responses, will interfere. A muscle that shows merely a trace of function may sometimes show no trace at all; at other times, much more than just a trace.

Special fields of therapeutic exercises require special measurements. Posture work, cerebral palsy work, etc., require a particular adaptation of the general measuring procedure, but these variations will be dealt with in their respective places.

REQUIREMENTS OF MUSCLE TESTING

The measurement and testing of muscle function has to meet a number of requirements if it is to be a regular, integral part of the follow-up treatment of patients. Unless the measurements are taken at regular intervals, in all cases, rational treatment will be handicapped. The most important requirements are:

(1) ***Simplicity:*** Measurements must avoid complication. It should be possible to take them easily and quickly, without undue loss of time.

(2) ***Completeness:*** Measurements should be complete. They should include all pertinent data.

(3) ***Selectivity:*** Measurements should not be too expansive. Every detail not of primary significance for the type of case should be omitted. See *Regional Testing* (*see* Figs. 44 and 9).

(4) ***Standardization:*** Measurements should be standardized.

While in this field we are still far from generally accepted standards, we are moving quickly in that direction. Meanwhile it is important to develop typical, standardized measurements in as many treatment centers as possible. Unless measurements are taken in identical manner, their value is obviously questionable. Findings obtained by different means cannot be compared. Without equivalent measurements, it will be impossible to follow a case quantitatively.

To sum up: The *purpose* of testing and measuring motor function is:
(1) To find a quantitative basis for an exercise program.
(2) To follow case development.

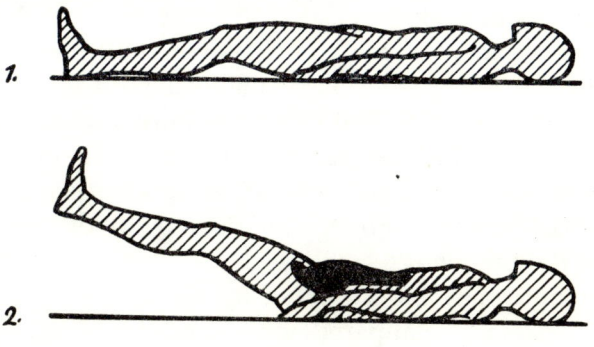

TESTING POWER OF "LOWER" ABDOMINAL MUSCLES

Fig. 9

There are a number of *approaches* to the measurement of muscle function and joint range. The following discussion will take up, consecutively, the measurement of muscle strength, muscle elasticity and coordination, and will briefly mention joint-range measurements.

MEASUREMENT OF MUSCLE STRENGTH

The most frequently used method of grading muscle strength is that which differentiates five (5) degrees of strength and zero (0), the complete absence of muscle contraction. Various authors and clinics use different variations of this procedure, which are, however, in principle the same. The scale runs as follows:

0 *No* voluntary contraction noticeable.
1 *Traces* of voluntary contraction noticeable.
2 *Poor* muscle power: muscle can produce movement if assisted and if gravity is eliminated.
3 *Fair* movement can be actively produced without assisance and against gravity.

4 *Good* as above, plus ability to overcome resistance, but less than normal.

5 *Normal.*

This method of grading is satisfactory if very weak muscles are graded (in neurological cases, infantile paralysis, etc.); it is inadequate if muscles between 4 and 5 are to be judged.

In numerous orthopedic cases, after fractures and injuries of all kinds, for instance, the weak muscles could all be classified as 4 (Good) in the 4-5 grade. They may all be able to take resistance and to lift weights, but only to a limited degree, and less than would be normal in comparable muscles of the same person. In such a case, grading must be further subdivided between 4 (Good) and 5 (Normal). For this, various methods are possible, among them the following:

(1) Strength may be estimated by the degree of resistance given to an extremity compared with normal and classified according to percentage of normal. Frequently 25% is taken as grade 1, and the muscles are graded from 1 to 4—4 being 100%.

(2) The lifting of weights, pulling or squeezing of springs, may be taken as the absolute value of muscle strength. Here it is hard to differentiate between one group and the next. The testing, while objective according to figures, will provide more general than specific information about the degree of muscle strength. It will represent a sort of performance or accomplishment test.

No matter which of these approaches is chosen, it will be important to establish comparable conditions when testing the same patient. Otherwise unequals are being compared. A few of the variables that may be excluded with care, are worth noting.

Momentary tiredness of muscle or lack of warm-up produce two opposed and entirely different conditions. A long walk, work, or previously performed exercises may tire or fatigue a muscle and cause relative weakness compared to that in previous tests. The same is true when the warm-up is incomplete or has not been performed. A muscle, when tested "cold," will usually show less strength.

If a muscle is tested by weight-lifting, the final weight lifted will be smaller than its maximum potential if this final weight has been found after a series of tries during which weight is increased (when the muscle has been tired by work). If this final weight is taken as a maximum strength potential, the mistake made will be magnified if the next test starts with the previously established "maximum" weight.

If repeated lifting of a weight, or the repetition of the same, equal strength performance, is tested, we are recording *endurance*. Endurance may be expressed by the number of identical performances repeated at short, equal intervals. Differences in speed and form will make the tests inaccurate or completely worthless.

The ability to hold a weight in one position, maintain a position against gravity, hold a spring, or, in other words, hold a contraction without movement, indicates *holding power*. The degree of holding power will be measured by the weight maintained and by the length of time the position can be held. The form of the movement or of the position held, the angle at which the test is made, and the joints involved, will permit conclusions as to what special muscle group plays a predominant part in the test.

Thorough knowledge of kinesiology is the basic requirement in helping determine the specific muscle group tested—and this is true of all phases of muscle testing. It is essential to stabilize to avoid substitution.

MEASUREMENT OF MUSCLE ELASTICITY

The maximum length of a muscle may be best gauged by measurement of the range of the joint—or joints—which it moves. Shortening of a muscle will restrict the range of this joint, or joints.

Joint range is usually measured with a *goniometer,* and the degree of the joint tested is compared with the range of normal joints. Joints of extremities are usually compared with corresponding joints on the other side of the body. When this is not feasible, in measuring trunk and neck motion comparison must be made with assumed normal figures.

It should be kept in mind that when joint ranges are measured, not only total length of muscles, but possible limitation of motion by pathology, is being measured: for instance, bone or joint deformities, shortening of joint capsules, loose joint-bodies,

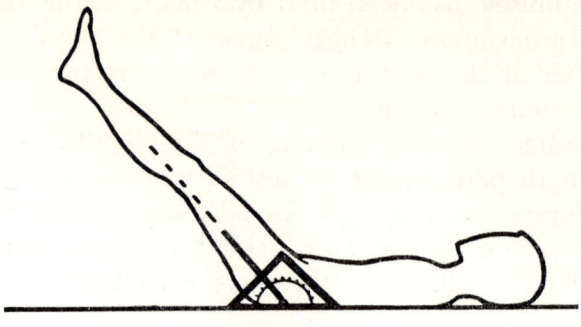

MEASURING HAMSTRING LENGTH

Fig. 10

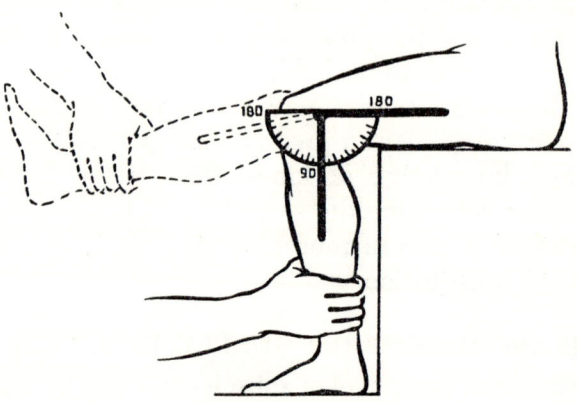

MEASURING JOINT RANGE (EXTENSION) OF KNEE WITH PROTRACTOR. CORRECT: LIMB SUPPORTED TO MEASURE RANGE INDEPENDENTLY OF MUSCLE-POWER.

Fig. 11

swelling intra- and extra-articular, adhesions, scars.

Some of these pathologies are readily seen or demonstrated by x-ray, and due allowance may be made for them. Others, such as capsular or pericapsular adhesions, can only be gauged by testing the joint range with the adjoining joints kept in varying positions. This will give the joint a chance to operate without muscular restriction. At least some of the possible restricting muscles can be eliminated by different positioning. If a gain of

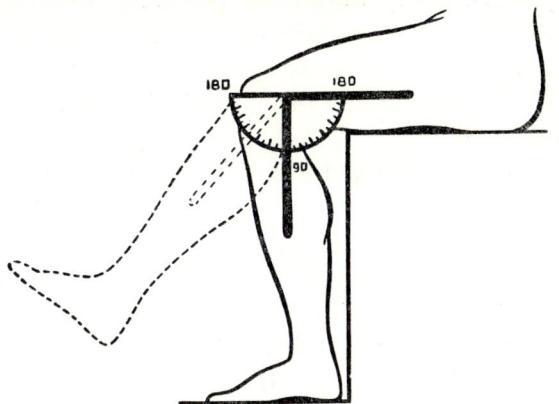

INCORRECT MEASURING AGAINST GRAVITY SHOWS SMALLER RANGE, INDICATES MUSCLE POWER RATHER THAN JOINT RANGE.

Fig. 12

joint range can be thus obtained, it may be concluded that limitations present are due to muscular (rather than other) pathology.

Again, as in the testing of muscle strength, tiredness and degree of warm-up must be taken into consideration. A tired muscle will often be foreshortened. A cold muscle will not extend to its maximum length.

Painful muscle spasm may be gauged by the limitation of joint motion. Increase of range obtained immediately after the use of surface anesthetics and exercises may help differentiate between limitation of motion due to spasm and limitation of motion due to contracture.

Spasticity (in upper motor neuron lesion) is usually graded by estimate: slight, +, and 2+ or 3+ spastic.*

Contracture is graded by range measurements as indicated at the beginning of this section. Allowance has to be made for spasticity or painful muscle spasm as well as for extraneous restrictions of movement and tension.

An important measurement, which is often neglected, is that for *increase of range* from cold to warmed-up muscle, and

---

* It is tested by placing a muscle in the most relaxed position, then rapidly trying to lengthen it. A spastic muscle opposes this with a quick jerking movement.

from actively warmed-up muscle to passively stretched muscle. The difference indicates the gain in elasticity through exercises. If the gain is large, proportionate improvement may be expected from exercises. If the increase of elasticity is small, the prognosis will be less favorable.

Tension may be gauged by passively lifting an extremity of a patient and requesting him to "let loose." A very tense patient will either anticipate the movement or will not "let go" and will keep the extremity elevated for a fraction of time before he actively relaxes the antigravity muscles causing the extremity to drop. When testing for general flexibility of back/hamstring muscles in a floor touch test, a stiff and tense patient will reach to a certain level from the floor only (Picture X-A). When made to relax his neck and his back, bending loosely from the hips and then made to reach down, he usually will gain a certain amount of inches (Picture X-B). The difference between these movements will give an appraisal of residual tension in respective muscles.—The adduction of shoulder blades, hunching of shoulders are other expressions of local tension.

MEASUREMENT OF COORDINATION

Measurement of coordination, or lack of it, is usually made with the aid of accomplishment tests. Note the number of failures in a given number of attempts. For instance:

Task (accomplishment): Touch nose with finger.

Failed seven out of ten tries.

Three failures out of ten tries will indicate improvement, etc. If desired, the number of accomplishments may be noted, instead of failures.

Sometimes the *length of time* during which positions can be maintained, or actions performed without failure, is registered.

The recording of time (minutes and seconds) is especially useful in measuring *"balance pictures."* Balance accomplishments that can be performed for short periods only, are considered to be improved if performance times increase. Once the task can be performed indefinitely, harder tasks may be given.

For example: sitting balance may be given, first with support. When this can be performed indefinitely, progress to sitting

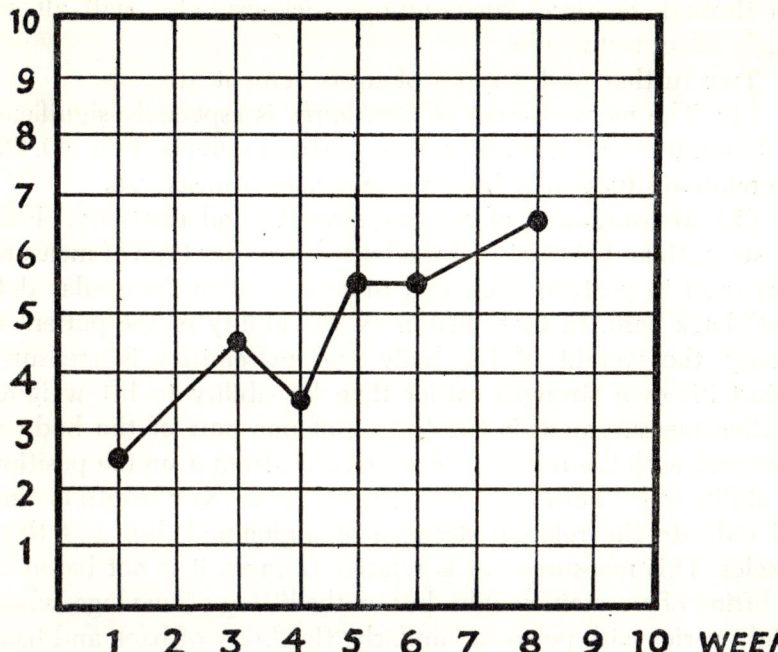

ACCOMPLISHMENT GRAPH:
TASK: TOUCH NOSE WITH FINGER,
NUMBER OF SUCCESSES IN 10 TRIES
TESTED ONCE A WEEK.

Fig. 13

balance without support. Then, successively, to: standing balance with support, standing balance without support, one-leg standing balance with support, one-leg standing balance without support, etc.

Time may be recorded by counting or by using a watch, stop-watch or metronome.

Involuntary motions may be gauged by recording the number of such motions occurring at rest in a given time unit or during given performances.

Again, it is important in the testing of coordination to establish equal testing conditions. Tiredness, emotional strain, distraction through changed surroundings, sickness, etc., will all adversely affect test results.

Two further useful types of measurement are:

(1) The measurement of *landmarks* is especially significant for deformities of the trunk, mainly postural defects (Figs. 40, 38). The relative situation of bony prominences is measured.

(2) Measurement of *relative* strength and elasticity. Relative strength and elasticity of the body is another type of measurement used in posture work and in treatment of "muscular deficient" back pain. In these instances, the ability of the patient to manage the weight of his body and extremities is measured against his own strength rather than his ability to lift weights. Relative measurement is the testing of one part of the body as compared with the rest of it. For instance, from a supine position, the ability to lift both legs to 30 degrees for a given length of time will indicate the relative strength of abdominal, hip and thigh muscles. This measurement is relative because it is not based on the lifting of a certain weight, but on the lifting of two legs, whose weight varies with persons. Similarly, flexibility of back and hamstring muscles in relation to body proportions is examined in the floor touch test. The above measurements, incidentally, illustrate the accomplishment test and, at the same time, a test for function of a whole body region—*regional function test* (*see* Figs. 44, 9). Accomplishment tests have been described in coordination measurements; they are especially important in lesion of the central nervous system. Regional function tests are important for testing and measuring large numbers of people for screening purposes.

RECORDING MEASUREMENTS

Measurements should be recorded identically, with special charts and measurement sheets for all cases. The charts will vary according to local requirements, based on the principles set forth in this chapter.

Results of repeated measurements will be used for graphs. Graphs, particularly useful when progress is slow and not obvious without careful recording, will give an immediate impression of the development of a case.

Recording of progress by charts or graphs will also be of great value in obtaining the patient's intelligent cooperation. Most patients will be stimulated by observing their progress, and will cooperate better when shown how much this progress depends on their own efforts.

RECOMMENDED READING

Daniels, L., Williams, M. and Worthingham, Catherine: *Muscle Testing and Techniques of Manual Examination.* Philadelphia & London, W. B. Saunders Co., 1946.

Duvall, Allan N., Houtz, Sarah Jane, and Hellebrand, F. A.: Reliability of a single effort muscle test. *Arch. Phys. Med.*, 28:No. 4, 213-218, April 1947.

Kraus, Hans: The indications of therapeutic exercises. East. Sect. Am. Congress of Phys. Med., 1951. *Therapy & Rehab.*, Dec. 1951.

———————————: Muscle testing in cerebral palsy. *Am. Phys. Therapy A.*, Feb. 1949.

Kraus, Hans and Eisenmenger-Weber, S.: Evaluation of posture based on structural and functional measurements. *Phys. Therapy Rev.*, 25: No. 6, Nov-Dec. 1945.

Lovett, Robert W.: *Treatment of Infantile Paralysis.* Philadelphia, P. Blackiston Son & Co., 1917.

Master, Arthur M. and Oppenheimer, E. T.: Simple exercise tolerance test for circulatory efficiency. *Am. J. M. Sc.*, 177:223-243, Feb. 1929.

Chapter 3

EXERCISE TECHNIQUES

EXERCISE TREATMENT AND THE TEACHING OF EXERCISES

IN OUR MECHANIZED society the majority of our patients have not had enough experience of physical exercise to develop good muscular response. Our patients are usually overtense, underexercised, reluctant to work their muscles and poorly coordinated. These patients will not readily do "home work" without going through a training period, and even after being sufficiently trained they can rarely be relied on to do exercises adequately, regularly and consistently when left to themselves. Therapeutic exercise sessions will therefore have to work in two ways:

(1) To "give" a treatment: to demonstrate the movements, to help the patient perform these movements, to give resistance; in other words, to treat the patient;

(2) To teach the patient, by explanation and direction, to do the exercises by himself.

The best possible results of treatment require that these two aspects receive equal attention.

Those exercises in which the therapist provides the major share of the moving power are called *passive exercises*. If the movement is performed entirely by the therapist, it constitutes a passive exercise, without further qualification.

If this passive exercise is performed within the present joint range without any forcing, it is a *gentle or relaxed passive exercise*. The value here may lie in the maintaining of joint range in case of paralysis—avoidance of contracture. If the patient has excessive muscle tension, and the passive exercise is performed with the patient keeping his muscles relaxed, its value is relaxation.

If the passive exercise is performed with a more or less gentle "push" or "pull" at the end of the range, with the purpose of overcoming contracture—of increasing joint range—the exercise is called a *passive stretch*.

A passive exercise performed with the patient's contributing power is a *passive-assistive exercise*. If the amount of strength contributed by the patient exceeds that contributed by the therapist, the exercise is called active-assistive. These two kinds of exercise vary in degree only, and their value may be both strength-building and relaxing. They lead to the next group of exercises, in which the patient's part is the larger, while the therapist acts as teacher.

A type of exercise in which patient and therapist have equal parts, is *resistive exercise*.

Resistive exercise is one in which the therapist opposes an attempted movement by the patient, or vice versa. The exercise value may be strength-building for the muscles overcoming resistance, that is, strength-building (mainly holding power) for the muscles resisting the therapist's pull. Resistive exercises may also be used to produce "reflex" relaxation for the antagonists of the contracting muscles.

Effectiveness of "reflex" relaxation can be demonstrated by having a person sit at the edge of a table and having him bent forward as much as possible. The person is then asked to extend his leg as high as he can and the degree of extension is measured. The same is repeated with resistance given to the leg, making the patient work his way up to maximum extension and gradually releasing resistance. This will result in increased extension.

Frequently, passive, assistive and resistive exercises need to be combined and used in one movement. Since the potential of strength and elasticity of different sectors of a joint range varies *(see Analysis)*, a single movement may require each one of the above exercises (Fig. 14). Starting with full passive, through help in passive-assistive, active-assistive, active, active-resistive movements and full-scale down to passive stretch again, every phase and dosage of these types of exercise may be necessary.

In rehabilitation of many orthopedic disabilities, peripheral nerve lesions, etc., this *combined assistive-resistive movement* may be the best, if not the only, means to give proper exercise value to every possible phase of joint range. This combined

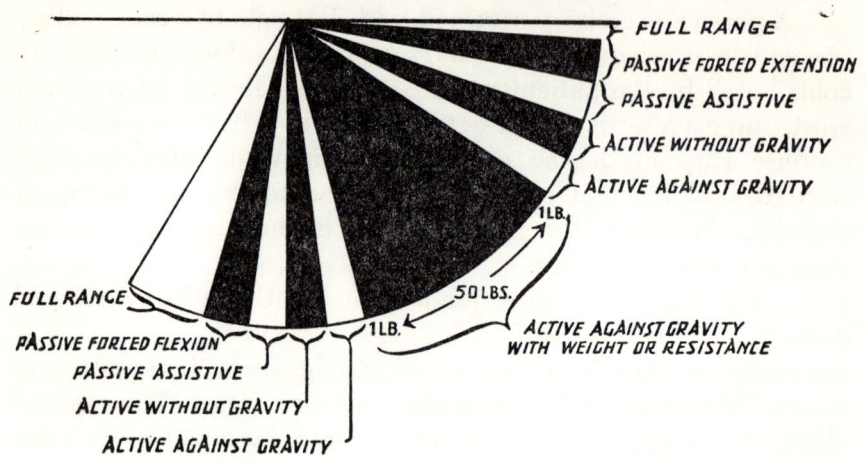

DIAGRAM ILLUSTRATING THAT DIFFERENT VALUES OF JOINT RANGE CAN BE ADEQUATELY COVERED ONLY BY MANUAL ASSISTANCE-RESISTANCE.

Fig. 14

movement cannot be duplicated by an exercise machine, which fails to cover all the phases in such a movement.

The therapist must be fully aware of the specific quality demanded for the different sectors of joint range. He should, moreover, accumulate enough experience to acquire a "touch" and "feel" for this kind of work, as an important and necessary addition to his knowledge.

Patients are expected, in the majority of cases, to do exercises daily, and this means only rarely in the presence of a therapist. Out-patients particularly must perform their daily exercises at home, either alone or with the help of a member of the family; the latter always holds true for children. Here appears the obvious importance of the *teaching aspect* of exercise treatment.

Successful teaching of exercises depends on certain rules:

(1) Exercises must be *simple*. Only uncomplicated movements can be properly understood by the patient. If a complicated movement is prescribed, it should be presented to the patient step by step, as it is built up from its elements.

(2) The *number of exercises* taught at any one session should be *small*. If the patient requires many exercises, limit the proportion of new ones introduced for homework, and make clear to the patient which exercises are to be done at home. In some cases, however, all the exercises may be included in the treatment.

Three exercises seem to be the maximum that can be successfully taught on one occasion. After the patient has learned quite a number, it may be advisable to add only one or two new exercises at a time. The patient ought to demonstrate *not enumerate* all his exercises at each treatment, in order to assume continuing proper execution. Written descriptions are sometimes helpful, especially in clinical circumstances, but mostly as a memorizing device. Verbal descriptions of exercises not only require special skill but frequently convey little to an untrained person; they are no substitute for actual performance.

(3) *Standardized presentation* of movements is effective. Any variation should either have a specific purpose or be avoided. The following routine is recommended:
  a. Starting position.
  b. Execution of movement to the point of its farthest deviation from the starting point.
  c. Return to starting position.
  d. Rest.

Rest should be mentioned as a definite phase of any exercise, since most patients are inclined to hurry.

(4) The movement should be not only described but demonstrated. The patient should then be guided or assisted when performing it for the first few times, always stabilized when necessary.

(5) The therapist, whenever possible, should base exercises on *pre-existing movement patterns*. It is much easier, for instance, for the patient to "raise his foot" than to "think of his anterior tibial muscle." It is much easier to make someone "touch his shoulder" than "contract his biceps" (*see* Fig. 79).

When the patient substitutes other muscles for the one that ought to be used, it is the therapist's job to devise an exercise that will make this substitution impossible. It is sometimes helpful to suggest "thinking" of a certain muscle, trying to pull at a demonstrated area, but such an approach should be considered a second choice if an easier one offers itself.

(6) Impress upon the patient the *importance* of doing the exercises and of doing them regularly. Sometimes it is helpful to explain the reason for a given exercise and for its execution in a particular way. It may be advisable to explain something about the main ideas of exercise therapy, etc. *Incentives* should be made clear to the patient and kept alive by the therapist. When neither understanding nor incentive is present, good results cannot be expected.

With young children such explanations are out of the question, and an entirely different approach will be necessary. Passive exercises should be given more extensively; conditioning and positioning exercises will have to be used.

Conditioning exercises are exercises in which rhythmic movements are passively performed, frequently to the tune of a simple song or nursery rhyme. The child learns to associate the same songs with the same movements and finally "takes over," that is, helps actively or actively performs what has been started as a merely passive movement. These conditioning exercises, may help to establish any of the three lacking qualities (*see* p. 5). They are a substitute for voluntary movements, and should be discarded as soon as voluntary exercises are possible.

Positioning exercises are substitutes for the volitional impulses by means of positional reflex. Holding a child's body in a certain position, for instance, flexing the pelvis over the edge of the treatment table, will cause reflex responses which are used mainly to work for muscle power.

(7) The *emotional state and mental capacity* of the patient must, of course, be taken into consideration.

BUILDING THE EXERCISE PERIOD

Exercise treatments should be built up from gentle and easy movements to more difficult and strenuous ones (Fig. 15). Start with an easy *warm-up;* increase in intensity to a *work-out* period, from which the main exercise-value will be derived; then decrease slowly through a cool-off period.

This pattern is easy to arrange, even in home exercises, once the patient has been taught to do his exercises in a certain sequence. To increase the exercises from easy to hard, and then to let the patient do the same ones in reverse, is the proper way to build an exercise "lesson" (*see* Fig. 15).

No muscle performs best immediately after a long rest; its qualities improve after relatively shorter or longer periods of exercise. To stop at the maximum point of work-out does not give the muscle an opportunity to return gradually to its resting state. These facts are known to all good athletic coaches, and should likewise be followed in therapeutic exercises.

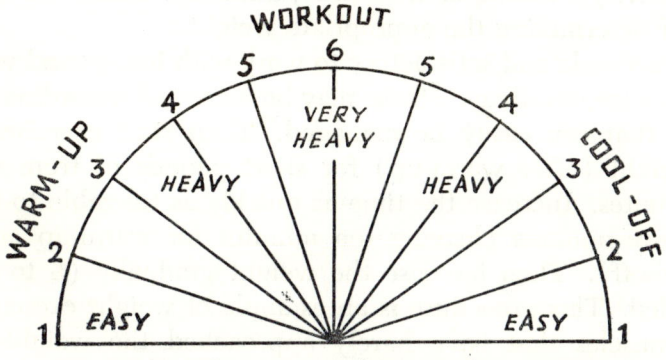

Fig. 15

EXERCISE TECHNIQUE

Exercise technique is the manner or form in which different types of exercises are used. These will be discussed in order of the established grouping: first, strength-building exercises, then elasticity development and finally exercises for co-ordination.

Strength-Building Exercises

(1) *Assistive* (active and passive) *exercises*. Here the therapist helps the patient perform the movement. This form of exercise grows out of lack of strength in the muscle to be exercised, which therefore requires assistance.

Assistance to the weak muscle may be given by other means:
 a. By the buoyance of water.
 b. By pulleys—operated by patient or therapist.

Assistive exercises have value as long as the muscle is too weak to perform satisfactorily in all phases, without help. Once the muscle is past this stage, once it is able to overcome gravity, begin the next group of strength-building exercises.

(2) **Exercises against gravity** require the lifting or moving of one part of an extremity or the trunk, without support. They can be graded by changing positions of arms, e.g., crossing arms in front of chest instead of holding them behind neck for sit-up exercises.

(3) **Weight exercises** are indicated for muscles that overcome gravity without, or with little, difficulty. There are various ways of determining the appropriate weight.

It is simple and satisfactory to work with half-pound weights (for instance, sandbags); these may be increased according to the weight that can easily be managed. Then start exercises with this weight (after warm-up) for short periods of from one to five minutes. Increase the time as quickly as tolerable to fifteen or twenty minutes (leaving ten minutes for warm-up and ten for cool-off). Then increase the weight gradually (½ to 1 lb.) as needed. This procedure is an example of weight exercises for weak muscles that have barely approached the weight-lifting stage.

Stronger muscles should be started on higher levels and may be worked up more rapidly. Any special method* using this approach may be successfully developed. Fatigue should, as a rule, be avoided. Fatigue (as defined by the training graph) produces a lessening of power lasting for at least a week, if maximum weights are continued. In real fatigue exercises, the total weight lifted will be smaller on the second than on the first day, and still smaller on the third and fourth days.

---

* DeLorme's Method: to increase the weight once a week, after testing the maximum weight that can be lifted 10 times—is helpful especially for clinical treatment of injured extremities. The 2 day rest period, given after the test days, is important.

Exercise Techniques   47

The same rules apply in the holding of weights for holding strength.

(4) *Resistive exercises,* which have already been discussed at length.

(5) *The use of a spring* for strength-building exercises has the disadvantage that the resistance offered by a spring increases as the opposing movement proceeds. This may be favorable in cases in which the maximum strength of the muscle is present in this final phase of movement (see diagram). It is a great disadvantage when this phase does not coincide with the more resistant phase of the spring.

Working against a spring should be used chiefly for strength-building of holding power.

(6) *Conditioning exercises,* (previously described) may be used as indirect approaches to strength-building exercises, which start when a child "takes over" and makes the active movement to which it has been conditioned.

(7) *Positioning exercises* for children provoke certain reflex movements by putting the child in certain positions (Fig. 19). For instance, the previously described hanging of the pelvis over the edge of the treatment table in supine position will cause contraction of abdominal muscles and double knee flexion.

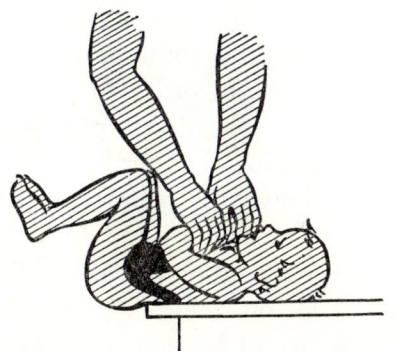

POSITIONING OVER EDGE OF TABLE TO
PROVOKE CONTRACTION OF ABDOMINAL
MUSCLES AND HIP FLEXORS

Fig. 16

Elasticity-Developing Exercises

To this group belong: (1) reflex relaxation; (2) assisted stretch and (3) passive stretch, which have already been described in detail. In addition there is (4) active stretch, which teaches the patient to contact the antagonists of the short muscle; this can sometimes be enhanced by resistance or weight to the antagonists (see reflex relaxation, Fig. 19).

(5) A constant, heavy *pull by traction or push by weights* placed over the contracted joint may be helpful only if no spasm or tension are present. (Fig. 20).

"Carrying weights in the hand" to overcome elbow flexion-contraction is not satisfactory. A weight heavy enough to overcome the elbow flexors is close to the borderline of the power of the finger flexors. Furthermore, the carrying of a weight in a hand tends to produce flexion of the elbow, since the superficial flexor of the fingers functions as flexor of the elbow as well.

"Pendulum" exercises, that is, the swinging of an arm when in a stooping position, may be helpful to improve relaxation in shoulder joints. To increase shoulder range, however, well-defined active or passive movements are usually preferable.

(6) The treatment of muscle spasm will be discussed in the following chapter on *management of pain.*

(7) Relaxation of the whole body or body regions is frequently needed in the treatment of our overtense patients. More often than not general relaxation training will have to precede the local training for relaxation. In order to produce general relaxation, the patient should be placed in supine position, made comfortable by placing a rolled towel under his neck and pillow under his knees. He is then shown the difference between tense and relaxed by asking him to tense a muscle, f.i. the biceps, and then relaxing it. Once the understanding for "relaxed" has been gained, the patient is asked to let go, relax, his arms, legs, his neck, his jaw, and he is made aware of tension when he does not comply with the request. Then he is asked to close his eyes, to inhale deeply through the nose and exhale slowly through tightened lips and concentrate in an attempt to let out his breath as regularly and slowly as possible. After each breath the patient should

Exercise Techniques

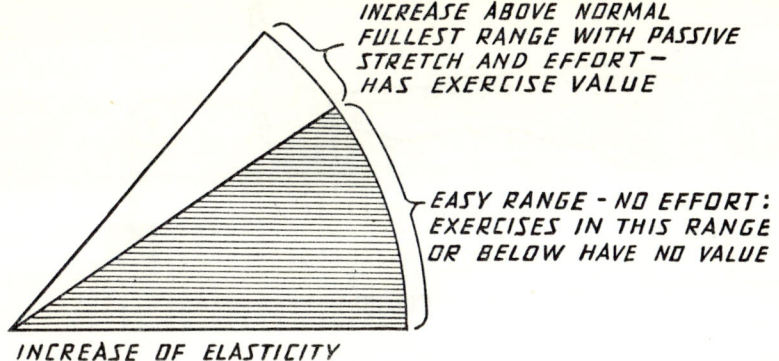

Fig. 17

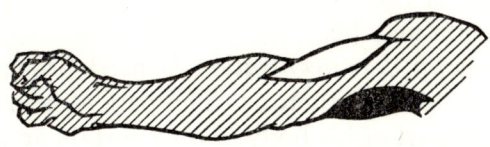

ACTIVE STRETCH BY ANTAGONIST
Fig. 18

REFLEX STRETCH FOR HAMSTRING

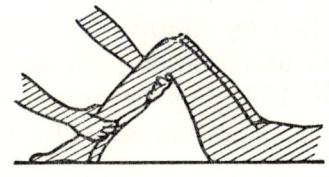

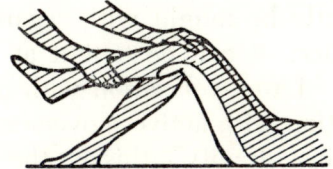

RESISTANCE GIVEN TO EXTENSORS OF KNEE
Fig. 19

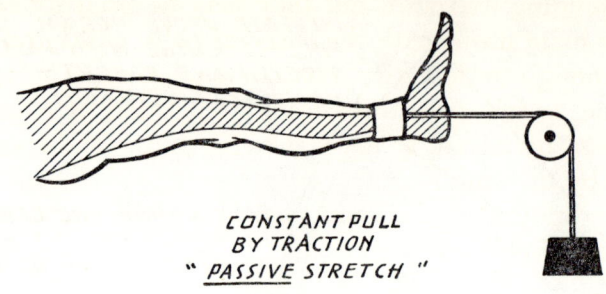

Fig. 20

again consciously let go and relax his extremities, neck muscles. This general relaxation will have to precede the local treatment in the management of the tension syndrome regardless where the target area of tension may be.

a. Relaxation *by deconcentration* is used primarily in the treatment of spasticity and athetosis. The patient is made to concentrate on another part of his body or on a certain action, usually breathing. He may be asked to fix his mind on certain thoughts, etc. A commonly used trick is the "Clench your fists and count to ten" trick, to make relaxation of the hamstrings and quadriceps possible when trying to elicit a patellar jerk. Marginal relaxation is the type of relaxation in which *some* of the attention is focussed on the movement and some on other regions of the body.

b. Direct relaxation *by contrast*: this type of relaxation described as part of general relaxation training starts by teaching the patient the difference in feeling between a tense and a relaxed muscle, through tensing a well muscle (for instance, the biceps) and then relaxing it.

After the feeling of tenseness is known, the feeling of relaxation may subsequently be taught with regard to one region of the body after another: it can be taught at rest, lying, sitting, and finally standing. Later, relaxation with passive movements, and still later, relaxation with active movements, will be learned.

Relaxation "against gravity"—this is, the suppressing of instinctive tensing when a passively raised arm is dropped—belongs to this group.

(8) **Conditioning exercises** have been described as

strength-building exercises, but they may be used for relaxation too. Their main use is with the cerebral palsy child until it is intelligent enough to do active, conscious relaxing. The technique is the same as for strength-building: repetition of a movement accompanied by a song to make possible active and spontaneous repetition by the child.

In the adult they are employed under the name of "habit-forming" exercises (*see* page 52).

Coordination Exercises

There are numerous cases characterized by defective coordination due to deficiency of strength or elasticity, or of both. When this is so, the first step in restoring coordination should be the restoration of the lost elements. Many other conditions require direct training in coordination, the most important being.
 a. Cases in which the elements cannot be restored.
 b. Central nervous system lesions leading to poor co-ordination.

(1) In cases with lost elements (i.e., qualities), it is necessary to try for *substitution* of the affected muscles by synergists, though in principle substitution of one or more muscles should be prevented as long as hope for return of normal function exists.

(2) The approach generally used in coordination exercises consists in breaking down complicated movement patterns into *simple patterns,* and in gradually building these up to a full, complex pattern. In this respect, the teaching of coordination is related to the teaching of skills. Teaching a patient how to make the best use of disabled extremities, and teaching the use of prostheses, belong in this group.

The group in which poor coordination is due to central nervous system lesions is treated principally by the same method. Simple tasks that can be accomplished are gradually developed to become more complicated; for instance, in ataxia (balance disturbance), simple "balance pictures" are gradually worked up to walking balance.

Athetosis *cannot* be treated by this method, since the superimposed involuntary movements are totally irregular. Repetition, as used to teach increasing tasks, fails, because each time the problem posed by the unvoluntary motion differs. Relaxation, elimination of the involuntary contraction should be used.

(3) *Conditioning exercises*, which have been dealt with earlier.

There is a final group to be mentioned in the teaching of coordination exercises, that is, the teaching of movement patterns, such as:

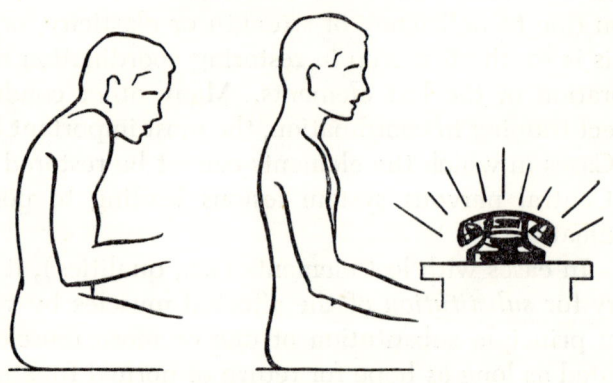

Fig. 21

(4) *Habit-forming exercises* (Fig. 21). An exercise is habit-forming if repeated frequently enough and persistently enough throughout the day to establish a "habit." Patients must be reminded of the importance of frequent repetition, which is sometimes achieved by keeping to a time schedule.

But for most adults it is better to combine the desired movement with an habitual event in the patient's life, to say, for instance: "Relax your shoulders every time your telephone rings."

Habit-forming should not be attempted before the proper muscular basis is present. It would be useless to say, "Hold yourself erect," unless the muscles were capable of sustaining this movement.

Habit-forming exercises are of special importance in posture work and in treatment of occupational strains.

GROUP WORK

All the techniques described are in principle the same, whether for the treatment of one or of more persons. The advantages of group work are competitive spirit and less likelihood of boredom.

If properly organized, students and fellow-patients may perform a helping role.

The main rules for organizing efficient group treatments are:

(1) Combine "equivalent or similar handicaps" only; knees with knees, etc.

(2) Subdivide the group into progressively increasing classes.

(3) Single out patients who require additional individual treatment and be sure that they receive it.

(4) Examine patients separately at regular and frequent intervals, and send them to more advanced classes as soon as possible.

(5) Separate groups according to age and sex.

EXERCISE APPARATUS

A great variety of exercise apparatus has been described by different authors. Some of these devices can be of help for certain special problems, and they may be necessary in dealing with large numbers of people. Very frequently they may be dispensed with in a normal exercise program or substituted for by simple aids, like sandbags, weights, etc. Rather than enter into descriptions of even the most well-known of these apparatuses, we refer interested readers to the bibliography.

Krusen, in *Physical Medicine,* gives a detailed survey of the most commonly used devices, with a comprehensive bibliography. Deaver gives a complete description of one of the most commonly used apparatus, pulley exercises.

One fact should be taken into account when using any of the numerous devices: It is often difficult to adapt a machine to the special requirements of a case. Before using a machine, there must be a thorough analysis of the requisite method or type of exercise and of all muscle groups thereby involved. All casual effects of an exercise machine should be studied carefully to avoid unpleasant surprises. Since even simple movements of the body are hard to define and analyze, and to reproduce in an identical way, complicated machines entail an especially meticulous exercise prescription.

Exercise machines never replace a good therapist. Giving of therapeutic exercises is a craft. The peresonal element, the "feel" of the therapist when giving assistive, resistive and passive exercises as well as his psychological effect cannot be duplicated by any apparatus.

RECOMMENDED READING

BILLIG-LOEWENDAHL, EVELYN: Mobilization of the Human Body. Los Angeles, The Billig Clinic.

DE LORME, THOMAS L. AND WATKINS, ARTHUR: Progressive Resistance Exercises. New York, Appleton Century Crofts, Inc., 1951.

HELLEBRANDT, F. A., PARISH, A. M. AND HOUTZ, S. J.: Influence of unilateral exercise on the contralateral limb. *Arch. Phys. Med.*, 28: No. 2, 76-85, Feb. 1947.

HELLEBRANDT, F. A.: Application of the overload principle to muscle training in man. *Am. J. Phys. Med.*, 37: No. 5, Oct. 1958.

JACOBSON, EDMUND: *Progressive Relaxation.* Chicago, Univ. Chicago Press, 1938.

KNOTT, MARGARET AND VOSS, DOROTHY: *Proprioceptive Neuromuscular Facilitation.* New York, Hoeber-Harper, 1956.

KRAUS, HANS AND EISENMENGER-WEBER, S.: Passive and active stretching of muscles. *Physiotherapy Rev.*, 1949.

PETERSON, FLEMMING AND BONDY: Muscle training by static concentric and eccentric contractions. *Acta phys. scandinav.* 48:Part 4, 406-416, 1960.

ZINEVIEFF, A. N.: Heavy resistance exercises: the "Oxford Technique." *Brit. J. Phys. Med.*, 14:6-129, June 1951. *Phys. Therapy Rev.*, 31: No. 12, Dec. 1951.

Chapter 4

TREATMENT OF PAIN AND PAINFUL MUSCLE SPASM

SINCE THIS BOOK is concerned with exercises, supportive measures, although desirable and sometimes important, will be mentioned only perfunctorily. An exception must be made in one large field: the management of pain, particularly, the management of pain in painful muscle spasm.

In the instance of muscle spasm, exercises without supportive treatment are almost always contra-indicated. Supportive treatment must first deal with the pain, in order to eliminate or decrease it to the point at which exercises can be performed without an increase of symptoms. A failure to understand the importance of pain in muscle spasm is responsible for many unsatisfactory results.

Definition

Painful muscle spasm is a clinical picture in which increased contraction of a muscle is associated with pain. The muscle is unable to give up a state of permanent contraction, and the result is painful limitation of motion. This disability of a muscle to give up contraction has been referred to in Chapter 2 as an impairment of the *physiological elasticity* of the muscle.

Painful muscle spasm can be caused by irritation or lesion of the central nervous system, by the muscle proper, joints, bones, or, in fact, of most of the tissues or organs of the body.

Painful muscle spasm is a frequent symptom of severe pathology. Should severe pathology be present, treatment of painful muscle spasm will have only palliative value, if any at all. Treatment of the cause is always preferable. In some conditions, we are unable to deal with the cause (e.g., poliomyelitis), or the cause may be only a minor or temporary irritation setting off the chain reflex of painful muscle spasm (as in cases of muscle strain or sprain). In the latter case, the symptomatic treatment of pain and muscle spasm may shorten suffering, restore normal motion and minimize or prevent the sequelae of muscle spasm.

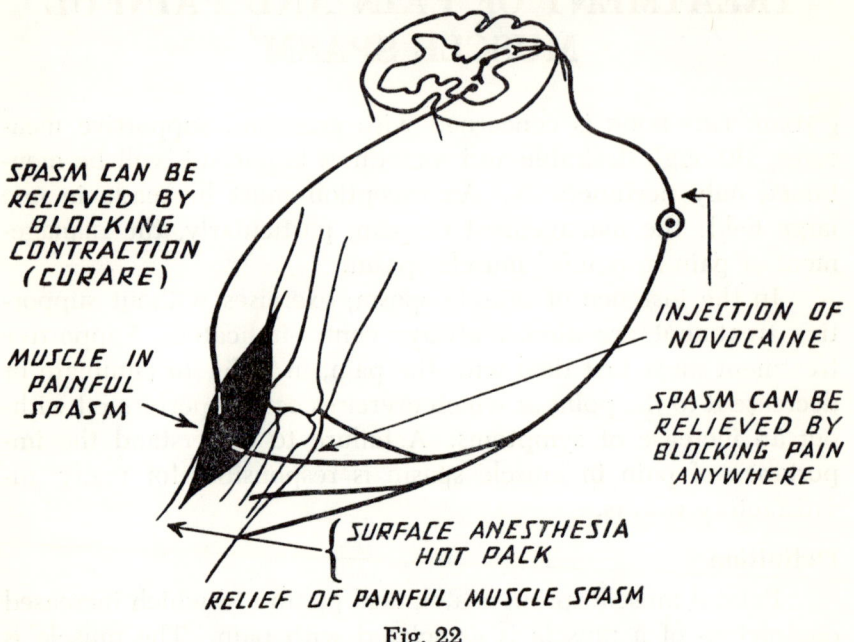

Fig. 22

In persistent painful muscle spasm, the muscle is contracted and frequently held in that state for a long time. Permanent loss of muscle elasticity and shortening, contracture are the most usual consequences.

Painful muscle spasm not to be confused with:

(1) *Spasticity due to upper motor neuron lesion* (*see* Fig. 8). No pain is present. The muscle reacts to a sudden pull with exaggerated stretch reflex (contraction). Relaxing and positioning in these cases frequently achieves complete relaxation.

(2) *Contracture:* A condition in which the muscle cannot be made to assume its normal length, but in which there is no pain unless violent stretching is done. The history will usually show a relative long duration. For treatment, *see* p. 48.

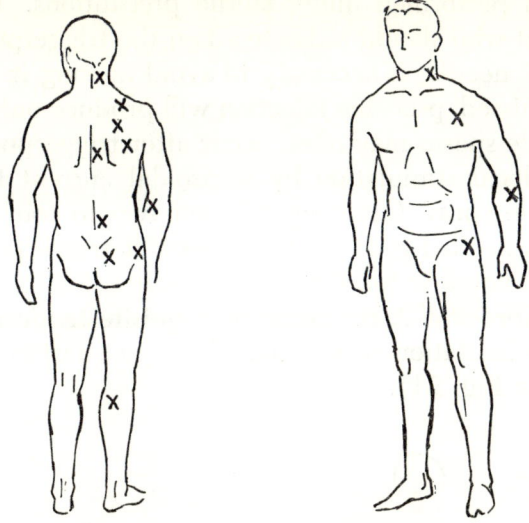

LOCATIONS OF TRIGGERPOINTS
Fig. 23

(3) **Triggerpoint** (*see* Fig. 23): The pain is located in small circumscribed areas of the muscle, exquisitely tender to touch.

These triggerpoints may cause local and radiating pain when a muscle is under tension or when minor strains or relative exertion of muscle occurs. Outside pressure, too, may trigger off attack of pain. Since triggerpoints can be activated by many different factors as long as they provoke muscle tension, spasm and contracture, these other causes may be held responsible. —Nerve root pressure by herniated disc, by narrowing intervertebral foramina, or by trauma may be blamed, when the origin of pain really was tension syndrome and a lack of physical outlet for emotional stimuli. —Careful palpation of the soft parts in every patient can detect these triggerpoints. In the acute attack they may be masked by muscle spasm. Treatment of triggerpoints consists of injection with procaine. Saline or even dry needling can be almost equally effective if properly done. The tender spot should be first located and marked on the skin, then the injection performed under sterile precautions. Cooperation of the patient who should indicate when the triggerpoint is penetrated by the needle, is necessary to avoid missing it. If the triggerpoint is missed, procaine injection will produce only temporary relief. Muscle spasm may often occur after triggerpoint injection and use of local stimulation by sinusoidal current followed by ethyl chloride spray (*see* page 62) on two to four subsequent days is often needed to avoid recurrence of triggerpoint. Use of hot packs at home is helpful.

(4) *Fibrositis:* A condition of exquisite tenderness of skin. It causes no limitation of motion. Therapy consists of pinching massage (*see* Fig. 24).

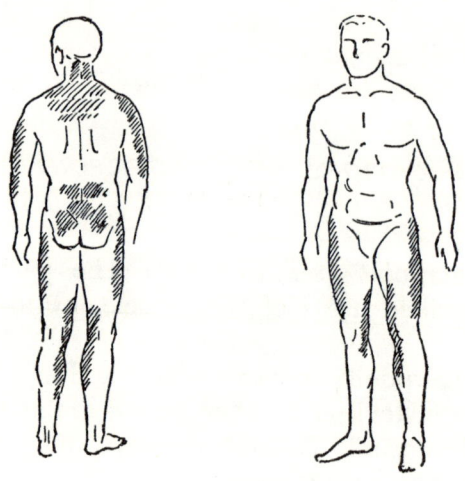

MOST FREQUENT SITE OF "FIBROSITIS"
SURFACE TENDERNESS
Fig. 24

(5) *Muscle Tension*: In his studies of bodily reactions to rage and fear Cannon emphasizes the necessity of discharging energies accumulated as preparation for fight and flight. When the individual is prevented from living out this response by using his readied muscles, tension remains. This muscle tension often results in physical discomfort.

Tiegel has shown that repeated tensing of a muscle results in loss of length in what he calls "Verkuerzungskontraktur" (contracture). This contracture and tension can be found frequently in persons subjected to chronic inhibition of the fight and flight response. There is a tremendous influx of stimuli to which the average sedentary city dweller is subjected. Traffic, telephone, high pressure work in the office or in school and competition in every phase of life all combine to keep us in a state of irritation. Seldom do we actually attack or run away, thus completing the action to which these various stimuli prepare our body and especially our striated muscle. We are forced by rules of conduct and the morals of our civilization to "grin and bear it." Here we will not discuss the other internal changes produced by this fight or flight response, nor will we discuss what these changes can do to the individual when not permitted to be purposefully used as foreseen in the biological background of human beings. We shall confine ourselves to the immediate effort on the striated muscle produced by the direct muscular response to stress.

If a muscle is still further shortened through added stimuli, tension will increase to spasm, and this spasm actually will produce considerable pain. This tension pain has been beautifully demonstrated by British workers. They subjected people who complained of occasional headaches or pain in different muscle groups to a tension-producing interview. At the same time they registered electromyographic response of these muscles and in control muscle groups in the same individuals. It was shown that while the controls remained at normal activity, the painful muscle responded to irritation with high activity spikes and reacted with pain when the activity had reached a certain level. The "target area" of muscular tension may vary. It may be found in the occipital and frontal muscles as tension headaches and in trapezius and rhomboid muscles as painful necks. In low back areas tension may be an important factor in producing pain of the muscular deficient back; less often those target areas can be found in the legs, thighs, arms, or any place where muscle groups are frustrated in an attempt to give outlet to motor stimuli. Posture, occupation, emotional background, habits and other factors may determine the target area.

Usually stiffness and a vague pain is felt in the first weeks, months or years of the onset. As tension is accumulated and the same area is hit repeatedly, the muscles lose the ability to relax. They become tighter and tenser, and painful episodes provoked by lesser and lesser stimuli occur more frequently. These stimuli can be extrinsic or intrinsic. They may be triggered off by merely trivial trauma. Where ever these stimuli originate, they can produce a physical tension syndrome and physical pain if their outlet through muscle action is inhibited. This pain is often not affected by muscle relaxants and by pain-relieving medication, especially not if very tensely contracted areas (Triggerpoints, Muskelhaerten, Myogelosis) have developed. These triggerpoints (they have been amply described in the literature) in turn, may cause radiating and local pain when the muscle is under tension, or when minor strains and relative exertion of muscle occurs. Kelgren has simulated the triggerpoint effect by injection of hypertonic saline into muscle fasciae and has been able to duplicate some of the typical triggerpoint pain patterns.

Outside pressure, too, may trigger off attack of pain. Frequently, these radiating pains suggest nerve root involvement. Since triggerpoints can be activated by many different factors as long as they provoke muscle tension, spasm, and contracture, these other causes may be held responsible. Nerve root pressure by a herniated disc, by narrowing intervertebral foramina, or by other trauma, may be blamed, when the origin of pain really was tension syndrome and a lack of physical outlet for emotional stimuli.

More frequently, tension combines with minor pathology setting up a vicious cycle, leading to considerable pain and disability.

A "nervous" individual caught in such a cycle, will look at his complaints through the magnifying glass of his own emotional disposition, thus compounding both pain and disability.

Once tension has progressed to the point of muscle spasm, treatment of pain and spasm itself will be necessary. This should soon be supplemented by relaxation training.

Common Treatment Principles

The treatment of painful muscle spasm observes a rule that is basic for exercise threatment *whenever pain is present,* and that demands:

Never pass the pain limit!

Never cause pain by movement!

The common principles of the treatment of painful muscle spasm in all procedures are: first, relieve the pain; second, start gentle movements to return the muscles to the normal length and relaxation.

There are various ways to attempt relief of pain and painful muscle spasm. Among those used in physical therapy—to which the discussion is limited here—are:

(1) The use of heat.
(2) The use of surface anesthetics.
(3) The use of surface "counter irritants," such as histamine iontophoresis.
(4) Use of tetanizing and sinusoidal current.

The use of pain-relieving sedative drugs and tranquilizers will frequently be indicated as accessory medication. The local use of novocaine injections has already been described. It should be reserved for Triggerpoints, *not* used in presence of muscle spasm.

The Use of Heat

(1) *Indication:* Acute painful muscle spasm, such as in acute strain. Irritation of lower motor neuron.

(2) *Contra-indication:* Any condition in which local increase of fluids (e.g., blood or lymph) must be avoided. Acute sprains and strains of muscles combined with local hemorrhage are therefore excluded.

(3) *Technique:* a. *Hot Packs:* Woollen cloths are soaked in boiling water, well wrung out and then applied to the painful area and covered with oil-cloth. They should be left as long as they remain hot (10-15 min.), then prepared and applied again. This should be repeated several times a day.

Towels may be used instead of woollen cloths, and dry towels, rubber sheets, etc., instead of oil-cloth.

The shape of the hot pack should be determined by the size of the painful area, but the exact shape is of secondary importance as long as the area is covered. While standardized packs are useful for clinical requirements, it is more important to apply the packs hot and quickly than in a standard manner.

b. *Local Hot Baths* for extremities (temperature up to 105°) may give relief if the limb can be placed in the container in a *comfortable* position.

c. *General Hot Baths* are helpful in more generalized painful muscle spasm. Again, the procedure must not cause discomfort through movements on the part of the patient.

The Use of Surface Anesthetics

(1) **Indication:** Painful muscle spasm. In the presence of major pathology, surface anesthetics may be used as symptomatic treatment. The decision of whether immobilization or surgery is needed, has to be weighed carefully. Immobilization or surgery will be needed if the structural changes present are too severe to be accepted or if increase by movement has to be feared. For example, in muscle strains and sprains immediate mobilization will be preferable, if major tears requiring repairs are not present. In fractures immediate mobilization may be possible if there is no displacement present or to be expected, or if the present displacement will not cause difficulty of function.

(2) **Technique:**

a. Use of *Ethyl Chloride* Spray*.

The painful region must be determined through active motion, but first of all, the direction in which the motion is impaired. Ethyl chloride is then sprayed on this area of skin. The patient then starts active motion of the part involved, in the direction in which motion has been painful and limited. As the pa-

---

*Kraus, Hans: Use of Ethyl Chloride Spray in Painful Limitation of Motion. *J.A.M.A., 116*:2582, June 7, 1941.

Kraus, Hans: New Treatment for Injured Joints. *J.A.M.A., 104*:1261, April 6, 1935.

tient carefully increases the movement, new painful areas—which up to this point have been concealed through limited motion—will develop. Those areas again have to be sprayed, and active motion continued.

These treatments last from ten to thirty minutes, and should be carried out with care and within the limits of pain.

Immediate normal use of the affected part may be allowed in the majority of cases, but excessive strain and sudden movement should be prohibited. Patients with more severe disorders should be prescribed rest, but all patients should be advised to continue the active movements that have been taught—from twice a day to once every hour—for approximately five minutes. While a single treatment will suffice in cases of minor involvement, patients with more serious difficulty will need more frequent treatment: during the first week, daily, and later, every other day.

An effective treatment should not require the anesthetic after the second week. Active motion will have to continue until normal muscular power is restored.

Immobilization after treatment is contrary to the basic principle.

Excessive use of ethyl chloride spray may result in frostbite of the skin. To prevent this, camphor liniment may be used. Avoid heat after use of the spray.

Active motion, though unquestionably necessary, should never be used brusquely or abruptly, in order to avoid injuries to painful spastic muscles, which would destroy the effect of the exercise.

Compared with the injection of procaine hydrochloride into the muscles and ligaments, the use of ethyl chloride in acute muscle spasm has these advantages: (1) Application is simple. (2) Repeated application is possible with less difficulty and risk. (3) Large areas can be controlled that would otherwise require vast quantities of procaine hydrochloride. (4) Ethyl chloride is ineffective when major fractures or tears are present, and is thus more selective and less dangerous. (5) It is better as a diagnostic means, since it is more selective. (6) There is less risk of a local after-effect, and there is no general after-effect, such as occurs sometimes after the administration of procaine hydrochloride. (7) There is no danger of infection.

Ethyl Chloride spray may be effective to relieve pain caused by triggerpoints but will not be effective to relieve triggerpoints proper. Injection will be necessary.

    b. *Novocaine Iontophoresis**

A solution of 1% novocaine hydrochloride and 1/20,000 adrenalin in 80% alcohol is used. Treatment area must be considerably larger than the one of pain distribution. A gauze pad of two to four layers is soaked in the solution and placed over the treatment area. A cotton crash towel, folded once or twice, soaked in saline, is then spread over the gauze, and a flexible, padded metal electrode is placed over it. This metal contact must be smaller than the area of the towel; and, above all, no metal should touch the patient's skin. The positive pole of a source of galvanic current is attached to the metal electrode. This combination electrode is carefully fixed in place with sandbags or bandages. A neutral electrode of approximately the same size, moistened with weak saline, is connected with the negative pole. The current is weakly applied and increased to 20 milliamperes and permitted to flow for 20 minutes. The current is then gently reduced to 0, and the electrodes are removed. The area treated usually shows blanching.

There will be surface analgesia, which will remain for approximately three to four hours over the area treated. This process makes possible the effective exercise treatment which is to follow. The analgesic effect lasts up to four hours. Except for the usual period of sleep, the patient continues to carry out the exercises at the regular prescribed intervals. Do not use local heat as long as effect of surface anesthetic is present.

The following rules must be observed for effective use of surface anesthetics (Ethyl Chloride or others): (1) The application must be made over an adequate area. (2) Do not use a too small indifferent electrode. (3) Application should only be made to a skin surface free of grease. (4) Avoid the use of dyed solutions which may produce a persistent coloration of the treated area. Use only pure chemicals. (5) Correct exercises must be

---

*Snow and Kraus: Novocaine Iontophoresis for Painful Limitation of Motion. *Mil. Surgeon,* 95:—, 5, Nov., 1944.

prescribed: not too rapid, not too strenuous and not too numerous. Exercises are to be given within pain limits. (6) Full instructions for the entire period between treatments must be given, consistent with the patients condition. These instructions should include a specific exercise routine which is a definite part of the treatment proper. Advise the patient to avoid influences that might ordinarily affect the treatment, that is make suggestions concerning the use of hard bed, firm mattress, proper chairs, correct shoes, rest (*see* Chapter 6). (7) The patient must be warned not to use hot applications over the area treated for at least an hour following the treatment; during this period the skin remains hyposensitive.

The administration of surface anesthesia is only the first step in the treatment of painful muscle spasm. Exercise is the necessary second step. Without it, the use of surface anesthesia would accomplish little more than the use of gas or ether in surgery without the surgical operation.

Exercises must be performed immediately after application of the anesthetic (with ethyl chloride, even while it is being applied). These should be exercises to *restore elasticity,* increase length and relaxation of the muscle (*see* Chapter 3), and should be given below pain and fatigue limits. Scattered dosage of from two to five minutes, and exercises every one-half to one hour should follow. The supportive prescription may call for particular or complete rest between exercises.

Recurrent trauma, bad postural or occupational habits or sports, are subjects that must be dealth with (*see* Chapter 6). It is important not to overlook the question of transportation for outpatients. Patients who live far away or with inadequate means of transportation to and from the clinic, should be hospitalized; otherwise this type of treatment should not be attempted.

The most common mistakes made in treatment with surface anesthetics and exercises are:
    a. Failure to cover the full painful area with anesthetic.
    b. Overdosage of violent exercise.
    c. Neglect of the pain limit.
    d. Neglect of home exercises.
    e. Neglect of supportive prescriptions (*see* Chapter 6).
    f. Neglect of follow-up treatments.

g. Failure to explain properly the procedure to the patient and to arouse the necessary cooperation.

h. Wrong indication.

Familiarity with the use of surface anesthetics and exercises will make of this procedure a valuable assistant in the differential diagnosis. It is worth repeating that ethyl chloride is the preferred agent for this purpose.

If the use of ethyl chloride is followed by satisfactory return of function and relief of pain, and no localized tenderness remains, it is possible to assume that pain and spasm are not due to major pathology. For instance, a sprain or strain may be assumed instead of a fracture, or muscle strain instead of a more serious condition of the back.

If ethyl chloride is unsuccessful, major pathology may be present, and it is wise to look for joint lesion, not demonstrable through x-ray, or major ligament tears. Other possible factors are: tissue tear, contracture, myogelosis (triggerpoints) or fibrositis. Chronic recurrent trauma (such as in occupational strain, postural strain, etc.) may be responsible.*

As to the theory involved: pain, originating in one portion of the sensory motor chain, leads to reflex muscular spasm and locking of joints. This sensory motor chain consists of the following elements: sensory nerve, nerve center, motor nerve, muscle and sensory nerve. Pain originating in the course of this chain leads to muscular spasm. The spasm is in itself painful, and leads to further spasm. Elimination of pain at any point in the chain results in the breaking of the chain and, therefore, in relaxation of the muscular spasm. This may be achieved directly by the injection of an anesthetic into the muscle, joint, ligament, sensory nerve or spinal cord.

If the pain-free interval is used to restore the muscle to normal function, the spasm does not recur, or it recurs with much less intensity. According to observation, on the basis of this chain, cutaneous anesthesia similarly relieves deep-seated pain in muscular spasm.

---

*Histamine iontophoresis has been found an efficient treatment for certain types of pain. Exercises, however, are not an integral part of its administration. It is, therefore, not discussed in detail.

There is no adequate explanation of the deep effect of surface anesthesia. It seems to be a fact, but the underlying physiological reason presents an interesting field for exploration. It must be definitely understood that surface anesthesia alone, without active motion, will not achieve good results.

Use of tentanizing and sinusoidal currents is another effective way to break acute painful muscle spasm. Electrodes are placed over most painful areas, e.g., both lumbo-sacral muscles or both gluteal muscles in low back pain. Tetanizing current is turned on gradually until good contraction of affected muscles has been obtained. Current should not exceed tolerance, should not be painful. It is left on for 10 minutes and then with the electrodes remaining in the same position, the current is turned off and sinusoidal current gradually applied until good contraction of the muscle is effected. Use of ethyl chloride spray and gentle limbering exercises following this procedure will frequently produce good results.

Evaluation of Pain in the Case History

Pain present when patient is moving a joint, and ceasing when at rest, is typical of injury or lesion of the joint proper, acute sprains, strains and fractures.

Pain after rest and improving with movement—jelling pain—is typical of "osteoarthritic" joints, improving or mild sprains and strains.

Pain upon weight-bearing is typical of "static" deficiencies or overstrain of the lower extremities.

Pain after work or while working may indicate an occupational factor.

Pain immediately after injury may denote a fracture or a major tear of muscle, ligament or tissue.

Pain after an interval is most often a consequence of minor strain or sprain.

Pain radiating along the distribution of a nerve may point towards radiculitis or mechanical root pressure.

Pressure by contracted muscles may cause pain of neurological distribution. —Pain caused by triggerpoints frequently has radiating character of typical distribution (*see* picture 23) and should not be confused with nerve pressure.

All these symptoms as related by the patient will never of themselves permit a diagnosis, but they may assist in arriving at one.

Since we have no real, practicable way to measure pain (devices that have been described are too complicated for general use), it has to be done by observation. It takes great experience to evaluate adequately patients' complaints.

In living up to the rule: "Respect the pain limit," you will frequently "undertreat" patients who profess to have pain when they are really experiencing the expectation of it. But it is part of the making of a good exercise therapist to know where pain starts and, therefore, where to stop treatment. Some patients dissimulate pain; they present an equal problem—in reverse.

Too much respect for pain is always preferable to disregard of it.

Therefore—*respect* pain.

RECOMMENDED READING

KELLGREN, J. M.: Observations on referred pain arising from muscles. *Clin. Sc.*, 3:175-180, 1937-38.

KELLY, MICHAEL: The nature of fibrositis. A study of the causation of the myalgic lesion (rheumatic, traumatic, infective). *Am. Rheumat. Dis. J.*, 69:77, 1946.

KRAUS, HANS: New treatment for injured joints. Abstract *J.A.M.A.*, 104:1261, April 6, 1935.

————: The use of surface anesthesia in the treatment of painful motion. *J.A.M.A.*, 116:2582, June 7, 1941.

LANGE, MAX: *Die Muskelhaerten (myogelosen)*. Muenchen, J. F. Lehmann Verlag, 1931.

MELZACK, RONALD: The perception of pain. *The Scientific American*, Feb. 1961.

SAINSBURY, P. AND GIBSON, J. G.: Symptoms of anxiety and tension and the accompanying physiological changes in the muscular system. *J. Neurol.*, (British) 17:216, August, 1954.

SNOW, WILLIAM B. AND KRAUS, HANS: Novocaine iontophoresis for painful limitation of motion. *Mil. Surgeon*, 95:No. 5, Nov. 1944.

TRAVELL, JANET: Mechanism of relief of pain in sprains by local injection techniques. *Fed. Proc. Cornell M. Co.*, 6:1:379, March 1947.

————: Ethyl chloride spray for painful muscle spasm. *Arch. Phys. Med.*, 33:291-298, May, 1952.

————: Trigger areas. *J.A.M.A.* 125:No. 7 adv., June 13, 1953.

Chapter 5

THE EXERCISE PRESCRIPTION

A WRITTEN EXERCISE prescription is necessary for record purposes. When two or more persons are involved in treating a patient, the prescription becomes an essential part of the treatment itself. It is useful for any or all of these individuals concerned: the physician, the surgeon, the physical therapy doctor, the head therapist and the therapist in charge of the patient.

The patient may have been referred simply "for exercises" which is equivalent to expressing an opinion that exercises are indicated. It does not, of course, constitute a prescription. **The prescription must be precise and definite.**

It is up to the person immediately in charge of physical therapy to write the detailed prescription. The referring surgeon or physician will frequently express special wishes (e.g., to abstain from certain movements, to abstain from weight-bearing, to emphasize strengthening, etc.), and these wishes should be carefully observed when writing the exercise prescription. When such wishes do not seem to fit into the total prescription, the referring physician and the therapist should confer in order to determine together the proper exercise treatment.

The exercise prescription will be valuable only if it comprehends or at least conveys: (1) the region to be exercised, (2) the exact type and form of exercises required, and (3) the dosage of exercise prescribed. No physician merely prescribes "medicine"; he always specifies both drug and exact dosage.

BODY REGION TO BE EXERCISED

Exercises may be prescribed for:
1. The whole body—total, general exercises.
2. Extremities—upper and lower respectively, or
3. Parts of the extremities—finger, foot, etc.

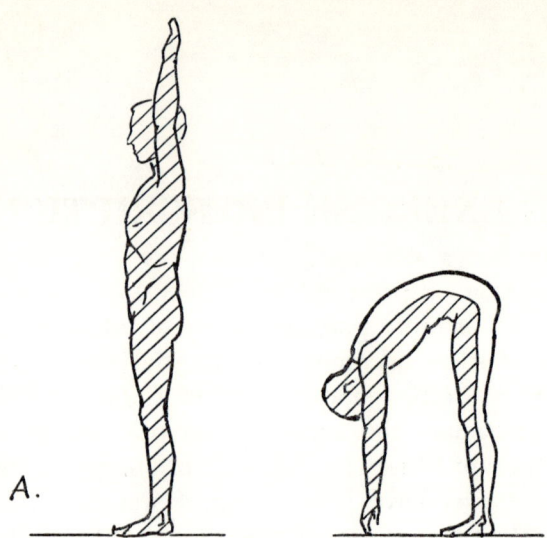

A. ILLUSTRATES: EXERCISE TO INCREASE ELASTICITY OF BACK, HAMSTRING AND CALF MUSCLES.

Fig. 25

4. Joints—hip, knee, shoulder, etc.
5. Muscles or muscle groups—flexors of elbows, quadriceps, etc.

The specifications chosen will depend on the individual requirements of the case. For example:

    a. A convalescent patient with no special weakness or disability will require "general" exercises.

    b. A totally weak lower extremity after injury, with both weakness and foreshortening of muscles present, will require "strength-building exercises and stretching exercises" with detailed specifications, such as "stress quadriceps strength" or "stretch calf muscles."

    c. Deficiencies of special muscle groups will call for exercises particularly affecting these muscles.

The Exercise Prescription

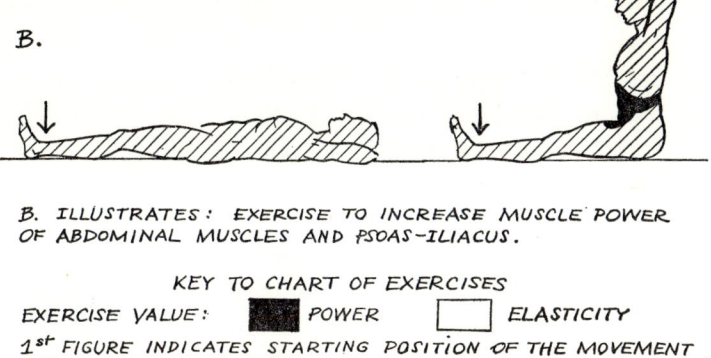

B. ILLUSTRATES: EXERCISE TO INCREASE MUSCLE POWER OF ABDOMINAL MUSCLES AND PSOAS-ILIACUS.

KEY TO CHART OF EXERCISES
EXERCISE VALUE: ■ POWER   □ ELASTICITY
1st FIGURE INDICATES STARTING POSITION OF THE MOVEMENT
2nd FIGURE INDICATES END POSITION.
(RETURN TO STARTING POSITION IS NOT INDICATED)

Fig. 26

EXACT TYPE AND FORM OF EXERCISES

The type of exercise prescribed depends on the quality that is to be developed.

If increase of muscle strength is desired, indicate this by noting down "strength-building exercises." Holding-power exercises must be mentioned if strength increase of this kind is required.

For elasticity, indicate in the prescription the special type, for instance:

    a. Stretching exercises: for contracture.
    b. Reflex relaxation exercises: for increase of physiological elasticity or contracture.
    c. Passive stretching: for contractures.
    d. Relaxation exercises, etc., as described in previous chapters, should be specifically mentioned.

Unless standardized exercises for typical cases have been previously agreed upon between the writer of the prescription and the therapist, it will be necessary to describe the movement desired and the form in which it should be executed. For example:

    Strength-building exercises for flexors of wrist: Place forearm on table, hand hanging over the edge. Flex against resistance. Keep fingers (a) stretched, (b) clinched.

Or another example:

Stretching exercises for hamstrings: passive stretching. Patient should lie supine. Passively raise leg with knee extended until stretch—not pain—is felt.

It is obvious that in a large clinic, or other working arrangement where many people have to be attended to this kind of detailed prescription is impossible. Prescriptions may be simplified by standardizing the form or movement of commonly used exercises. It will then only be necessary to prescribe a certain movement or to ask for a certain type of exercise; the therapist will understand exactly what is wanted.

To illustrate this simplified procedure, take the above prescription of strength-building for the wrist. The same results, in terms of actual treatment, could be obtained by stating simply "strength-building for wrist flexors," if the therapist is familiar with the approach desired. In the prescription "flex wrist against resistance," the *movement* is indicated, and the *quality* desired is expressed by the request for *resistance*. The form of the exercise has been standardized and need not be mentioned in so many words.

The fundamentals of form, such as slowness or movement, rest between movements, etc., must also be standardized in order to make possible rational treatments and prescriptions. This standardization can be achieved only if the person prescribing is thoroughly informed of the exercise techniques of the therapist giving the exercises. To this end, conferences, frequent comparing of notes, instructions and demonstrations will be necessary.

"Standardization" does not mean an established, fixed procedure. It means rather a common understanding and a common procedure. And the procedure must be flexible. Exercises should be changed in form and type if that is expedient, but changes should always be made in co-operation with all persons involved in the treatment. Otherwise the prescription itself will deteriorate into a useless gesture.

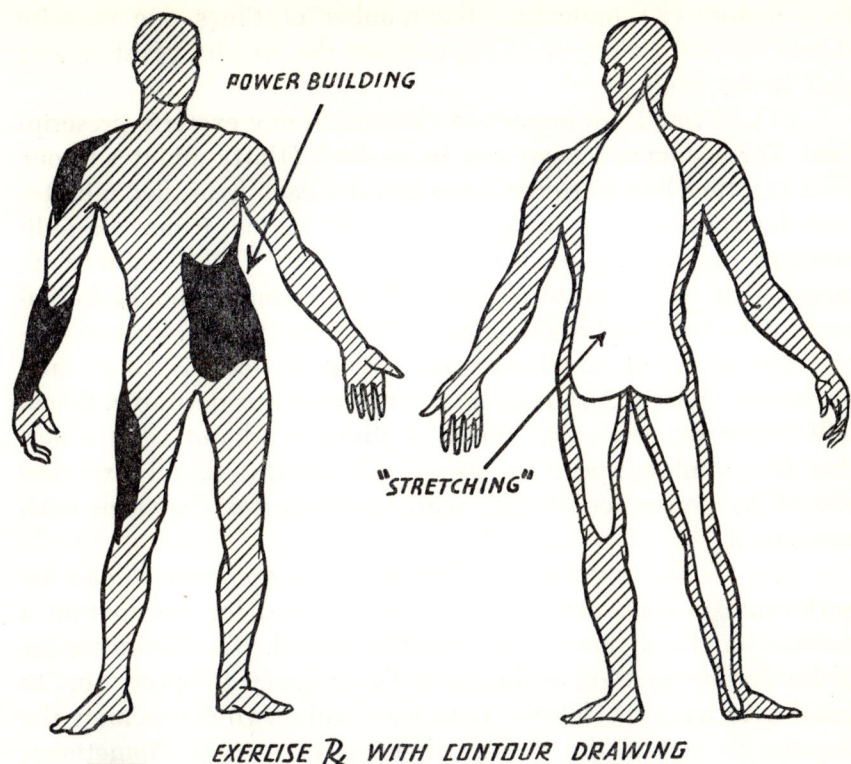

EXERCISE ℞ WITH CONTOUR DRAWING ▪ INDICATES POWER BUILDING. ☐ INDICATES ELASTICITY INCREASING (QUALIFICATIONS ADDED)

Fig. 27

PRESCRIPTION OF DOSAGE

Here, once again, exact prescription is most important.

If understanding among all the members of the physical therapy team is well-founded, the prescription of dosage need not be in great detail. Notations such as "keep below fatigue limit," "reach fatigue limit," "stretch—gentle—to pain limit," etc., will suffice. However, it is always better to be perhaps too detailed than to run the risk of omitting any phase of the dosage prescription

Dosage of exercise can be prescribed by: (1) noting the

time factor; (2) indicating the number of times one exercise should be performed; or (3) specifying the weight, resistance or pull to be used.

(1) *Time* is an important element in any exercise prescription. For instance, dosage may be *massive* (thirty minutes to one hour at a time) or *scattered* (two minutes each hour, five minutes each hour, etc.). If a gradual increase is desired, it may be indicated by drawing an arrow (10 min. x 2 $\xrightarrow{1 \text{ week}}$ 30 min. x 2, means that two exercise periods of ten minutes should be increased to two thirty-minute periods in one week).

The speed at which exercises are performed is an equally important matter. As a rule, a slow movement is desirable. Speed will rarely be perscribed unless a strong work-out is in order; therefore, unless speed is specifically indicated, all exercises should be performed slowly, with adequate rest between each movement.

(2) *Indicating the number of times exercises should be performed in each period* may be substituted for designating a definite length of time for the exercise period. The disadvantage of the former method is the patient's tendency to speed up, "to get it over with." A definite time limit laid down counteracts the impulse to exceed the desired slowness of motion. Sometimes, however, when very few movements at a time are to be executed, it is advisable to designate the number of performances; for instance: "flex/extend elbow three times every half-hour (3 x ½ hr.)."

(3) *The amount of intensity* for strength-building exercises may be prescribed by specifying the weight to be lifted or the resistance to be given (see Strength-building Exercises — Techniques). Weight may be expressed in pounds to be lifted or held. Resistance is usually expressed by requests for heavy, moderate or little resistance. Prescribing exercises with assistance, without gravity, against gravity, and finally with weight or against resistance, is the simplest way to grade power-building exercises.

Stretching of contractures is graded by notations as to gentle, moderate or strong passive stretching. Stretching by pull of the antagonist is usually not graded but done to capacity, the only grading factor being the time limit.

It is sometimes useful to add a general outline of the treatment program to the individual prescription.

Dosage of co-ordination exercises may be indicated by prescribing lengths of exercise periods. Here the dosage is greatly dependent on the attention span, co-operation, interest, etc., of the patient, and will vary from one time to another. A certain maximum for an exercise period should be decided upon and stated.

The most common mistakes in the writing of exercise prescriptions are:

(1) Prescribing "exercises," without further qualifications. This is *not* a prescription, it is merely a statement that the patient is suitable for exercise treatment.

(2) Failure to indicate exercise type or quality; omission of dosage.

(3) Lack of co-ordination or understanding between the person writing the prescription and the therapist.

To give an example of a prescription based on good co-ordination between those two persons, but not carried to full detail:

The problem: Left hemiplegia with spasticity, weakness and contractures of left upper and lower extremity. Disability: cannot walk, cannot use hand.

Ultimate aim: Use of left hand as assisting hand. Walking with cane, without brace (walking without cane seems unlikely in this fictitious case).

Immediate aim: Relaxation of both extremities and stretching of contractures.

Later: Strengthening of weak muscles.
Co-ordination.
Walking.
Occupational therapy.

Rx: *Relaxation* lying for both extremities: a) without movement; b) with passive movement; c) with assisted movement.

In b) and c) Upper extremity: flex/extend
elbow, finger
Lower extremity: flex/extend
ankle, knee, hip

Stretching for contractures (see Muscle Chart) passive, mild.

Strength-building (later) for weak muscles (see chart).

Duration of treatment: 15 min. $\xrightarrow{2 \text{ weeks}}$ 30 min.

Once the aims are outlined, the whole exercise procedure will be reasonably clear to all concerned. When the aim is obvious, the outline may, of course, be omitted; otherwise it will be a positive addition to the prescription.

It is important to remember that in many cases exercises will only be one part of the overall rehabilitition program. It will be necessary to coordinate therapeutic exercises with the other procedures. Care for mental or emotional difficulties, vocational and social adjustment and of course medical and surgical problems have to be considered before writing an exercise program.

Chapter 6

SUPPORTIVE PRESCRIPTIONS
(and other additions to the treatment)

FREQUENTLY EXERCISES are only one of two or more modalities of the physical therapy prescription. Medicine, diet, psychotherapy and occupational therapy may also be indicated for the same case. These additional prescriptions should not be neglected.

Additional treatment for special cases will be covered in chapters devoted to these matters. The treatment of pain, in which the additional therapy equals and sometimes exceeds in importance the exercises proper, has already been described. The present pages will take up certain phases of treatment by exercises, the influence exerted by the daily routine, occupational habits, games and athletic activities—all of which necessitate repeated, often standardized movements that may easily work against the exercise program.

The effectiveness of therapeutic exercises depends on sufficient repetition of standardized movements. If the daily habits that produced standardized movements and positions counteract the movements assigned in the program, the exercises may well be quite futile. This consequence is especially likely in treating conditions caused by faulty movement habits, such as many occupational and athletic-muscle conditions and many postural or other orthopedic conditions.

It is impossible to give more than a brief outline of the various typical movement patterns present in different phases of occupation, sport and daily habits. The following notes are offered as a lead, and not as a complete survey or even listing.

CLOTHING HABITS

Wearing the wrong clothes is responsible for many constantly repeated faulty movements:

(1) **Shoes:** Modern footwear—and this is especially true of women's shoes—is very unsatisfactory from the point of view of normal, physiological body mechanics. High heels are conductive to poor posture, foreshortened calf muscles and hamstrings and excessive weight-bearing on the forefoot. Narrow toes produce rigidity of the foot. If the inner contour of the shoe is not straight, it will produce hallux valgue; contractures of foot muscles. The foot will then work like a hoof instead of a grasping hand. Loose-fitting heels, "sling" heels and excessively narrow heels will

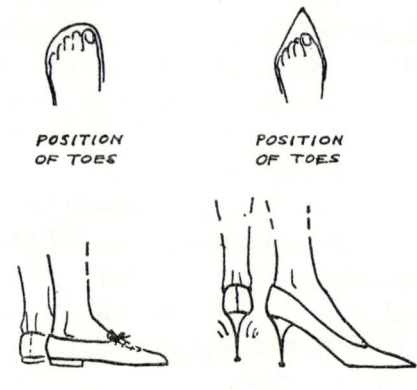

GOOD SHOES AND BAD SHOES

Fig. 28

produce swaying of the ankles at each step, with resulting chronic traumatization of the ankle joints and the long foot muscles. Knees, hip joints and back can all be affected by these artificially poor body mechanics and resulting inadequate movement patterns. Standing in such shoes may aggravate bad standing habits, such as constantly favoring one foot to relieve the other from a pinching shoe (see Fig. 28).

(2) **Stockings** are sometimes too tight, particularly around the toes, and may thus interfere with normal movements of toes and foot.

(3) **Girdles** may be too tight and may completely hinder trunk movements. They may turn bending into a caricature of the normal.

(4) **Brassieres**, especially those with very narrow straps, may contribute to painful shoulders and of pain in the upper back, partly by direct pressure, partly by forcing the wearer into a rigid posture of shoulders and back.

(5) **Collars** may prevent normal back movements when too tight or too high, and can cause stiff neck.

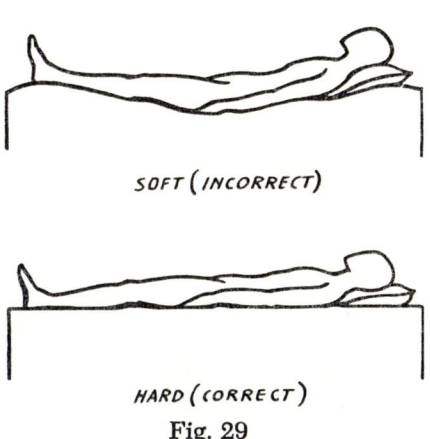

Fig. 29

Mattresses are frequently too soft (*see* Fig. 29). They should be firm, without inner springs, should not give or sag and should not hold the body in a groove preventing it from turning freely during sleep. Horsehair mattress on a board are generally the best. Sleeping positions are important, as regards not only the back but the neck and shoulders as well. The habit of sleeping with an arm in maximal abduction, or in a cramped position underneath the body, may be a contributing cause of shoulder and neck pain and may even affect circulation of the whole upper extremity. Similar complaints may arise from sleeping with too large or too small a pillow, the latter being especially inadvisable for people with broad shoulders (*see* Fig. 30). Reading in bed in a cramped position, draft, or uncovering part of the body during the night are all possible causes or aggravating symptoms.

Bending the back alone instead of bending with the knees, that is, bending incorrectly, is a frequent cause of backache. A

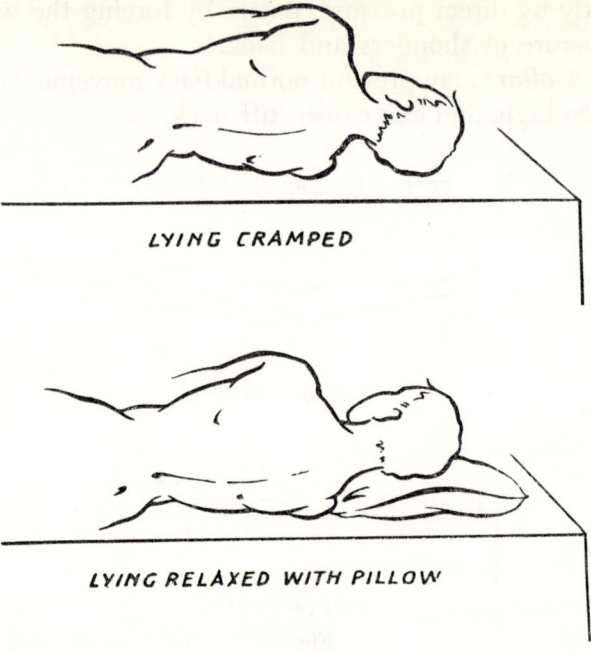

Fig. 30

strong flexible back in a well coordinated person does not require favoring. When this person is called on to lift excessive weights, he will instinctively use his body adequately and with proper posture. People with relatively weak and stiff backs will have to watch their lifting posture constantly and consciously. Stooping, one of the most common movements in household activities, can help produce pain (*see* Fig. 31). A patient asked to record the most necessary household details (outside of cleaning and making beds) arrived at a figure of close to one hundred with a single day.

Sweeping, carrying market baskets, turning door knobs, doing laundry and, even more, ironing, are all hazards which may produce pain in shoulders, elbows, wrists and back. Back pain particularly is often caused by making beds, opening windows and care of infants. Low cribs and growing babies are a combina-

Supportive Prescriptions

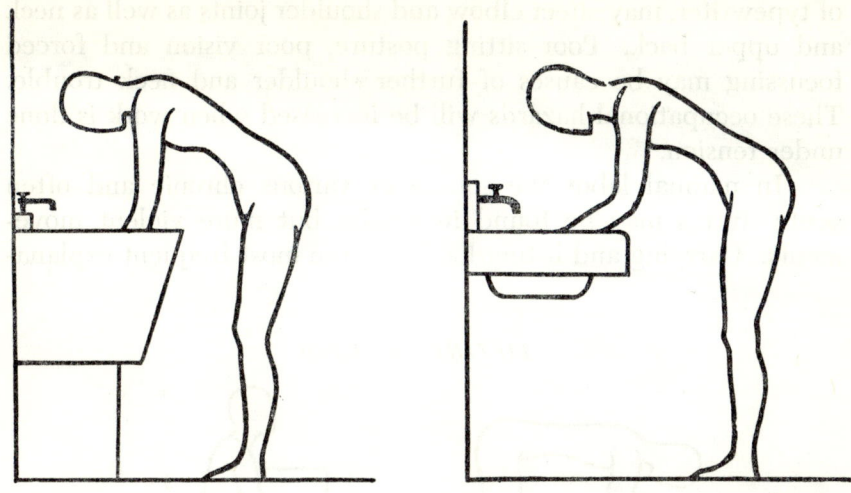

LOW BASIN AS A CAUSE OF BACK STRAIN

Fig. 31

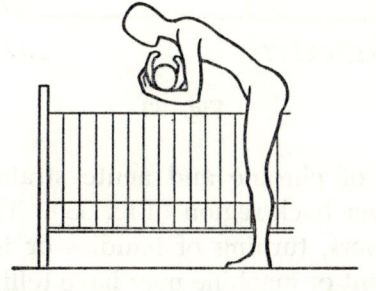

A LOW CRIB AS A CAUSE OF BACK STRAIN

Fig. 32

tion very damaging for many weakened mothers whose abdominal and back muscles are not prepared for the job (*see* Fig. 32).

WORKING HAZARDS

Even in apparently inconsequential office work there are numerous standardized movements and positions that may contribute to muscular and joint pain. Constant handling of the telephone, typing or writing with tense shoulders, awkward position of typewriter, may affect elbow and shoulder joints as well as neck and upper back. Poor sitting posture, poor vision and forced focussing may be causes of further shoulder and neck trouble. These occupational hazards will be increased when work is done under tension.

In manual labor the source of various chronic and often acute strains may be found in similar but more violent movements. Carrying and lifting loads are the most frequent explana-

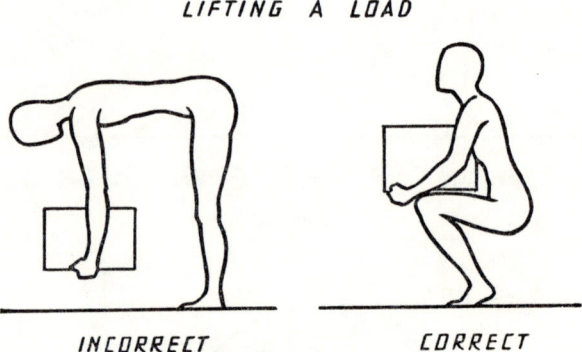

Fig. 33

tion for all sorts of chronic and acute strain, most commonly located in the lower back region (Fig. 33). The constant handling of elevator doors, turning of handles or identical use of almost any instrument or machine may have telling effects. Shoveling and the use of heavy hammers, especially when the blow hits a hard surface, may cause all sorts of strain of the upper extremity and shoulders.

All these detrimental effects are especially likely if work is performed by people who are not physically up to it, or if the same kind of work is performed without any variation of routine.

An unsolved problem arises from the return of workers to the same job that caused the disability. Much more attention should be paid to this, and to providing special training or rehabilitation jobs for people whose difficulties have been caused or aggravated by chronic, standardized movement patterns.

CHILDHOOD PATTERNS

All the bad influences of movements and positions repeated faultily are doubly significant in childhood, when not merely immediate discomfort and pain may result. The formative influence of muscle action may be conducive to postural deficiencies and permanent damage. No posture treatment should be attempted without carefully observing sitting habits, school desks, eye correction, ways of carrying schoolbooks (Figs. 34-36), athletic activities and, finally, adequate beds and mattresses. (This subject is dealt with more fully in the chapter on posture.) In our mechanized society our children are frequently underexercised and over-fed. They frequently fail to meet minimum muscle fitness standards.

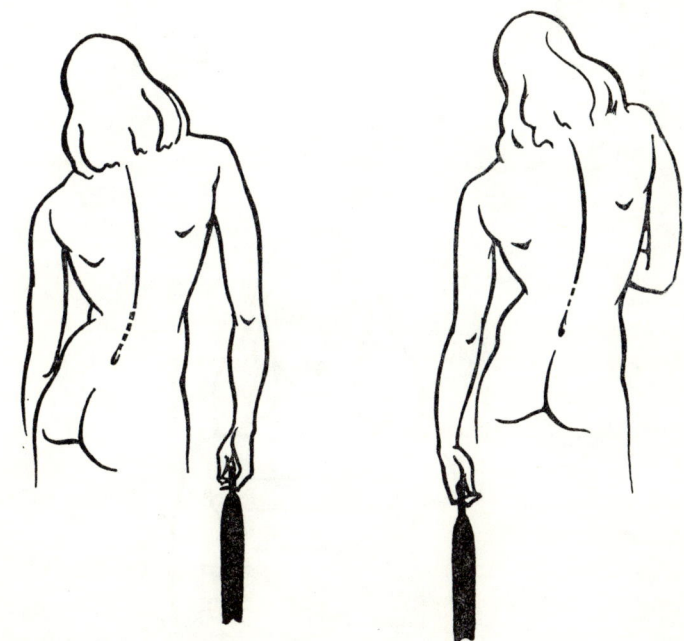

CARRYING BRIEFCASE, AS CAUSE OF POOR POSTURE

Fig. 34

ATHLETIC ACTIVITIES

Athletic injuries—both acute and chronic—form a large,

CARRYING BOOKS AS A CAUSE OF POOR POSTURE

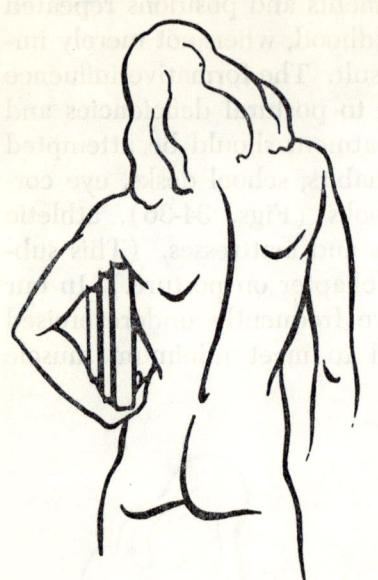
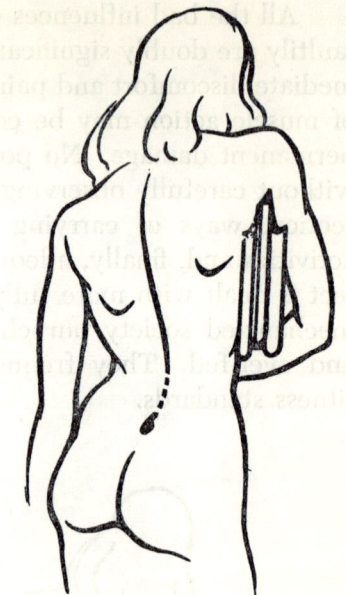

Fig. 35

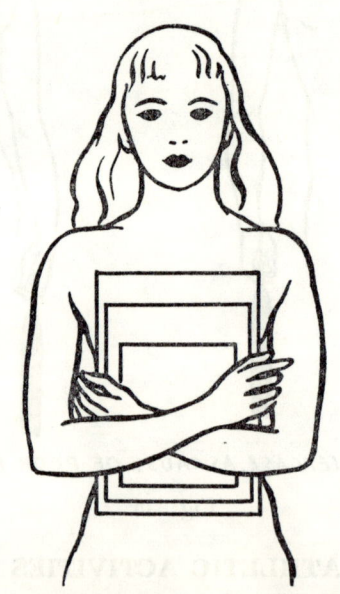

CORRECT WAY TO CARRY
SCHOOL PACK

Fig. 36

special field. Their treatment requires understanding of the movement that caused the injury, particularly the chronic one.

Since the damaging movement will be repeated constantly, as long as the sport is continued, it may often be necessary to stop the activity concerned. This is difficult, sometimes impossible. If the sport is professional or semi-professional, it will be necessary sooner or later to return to it. Changes in the "form" of the movement, minor changes in equipment, advice about warm-up and cool-off, etc., will be required to achieve even limited success in such cases.

If athletic activities are merely a diversion, it will be possible to abandon them. This, however, must be regarded as a failure to attain the main objective of exercise therapy: restitution of full use of the body.

Several examples of common sport problems are worth outlining here:

(1) *Track and Field:* Running, especially on hard tracks, may cause "split shins," pain in the anterior tibial region, which may frequently be relieved by shifting the weight-bearing surface of the foot by means of a metatarsal pad or by providing a softer track. Strain of the hamstring muscles is a common occurence in sprints—80- to 100-yard dashes. This strain can often be avoided by sufficient warm-up to make the hamstrings elastic enough for performance.

(2) *Javelin throwing* may produce painful shoulders and elbows, which are often relieved by minor changes in form or sufficient warm-up.

(3) *Baseball:* The baseball shoulder is a well-known athletic injury based on chronic, repeated, intense performance. Minor changes in form (if possible) and sufficient warm-up may be of help.

(4) *Tennis:* So-called "tennis elbow" may be caused by a topspin in the serve, by an incorrect backhand or by too small or too wide a racket handle.

(5) *Golf* may affect wrists, elbows and shoulders and likewise the back; it may also affect the pivot leg.

(6) *Swimming:* The crawl stroke may affect shoulders after an injury, and the breast stroke is frequently felt in the knees, after any injury.

(7) *Football, basketball and other ball games* contribute to a variety of less typical injuries. They may be caused by all sorts of movements or performances that are less standardized than in other sports.

(8) *Rowing,* especially sculling, can have a marked influence on posture; one-oared rowing particularly so. Exchanging port and starboard oars may effect unilateral asymmetries of spine and shoulder girdle.

(9) *Skating* may produce foot strain in weak feet, but may also be good for ankles and feet that are strong enough for the strain.

(10) *Skiing* produces very similar strain on the lower extremities, especially noticeable in incompletely compensated knee and ankle injuries.

An important preventive of athletic injuries to make the sport useful and enjoyable is general conditioning exercises. The respective athlete should first be in good general conditioning and perfect muscular shape before endulging in sports.

THE PATIENT'S ATTITUDE

The attitude of the patient may make the difference between success or failure of exercise therapy. Since the patient must of necessity cooperate in the program, he cannot be treated if he does not do so. It is best to inform the patient of the effort and time needed to produce worthwhile results and to make it clear to him that he has to do the work and nobody can do it for him. In children as well as in adults it will be necessary to exert a certain amount of discipline and firmness.

Our muscles are our only means of expressing what is in our mind. Our mind, subject to chronic irritation, finds its outlet many times in "tensing" one or more parts of the body. Tension will more often than not be part of the problem to be overcome when giving therapeutic exercises. Reassurances, relaxation training, explaining of the cause of tension, special instructions for changes of daily activities and posture, habit forming exercises wil have to be used.

A final consideration is the patient's place of residence. If the patient has to travel for an hour back and fourth in a subway, streetcar, or cramped in an automobile, in order to receive a treatment for, let us say, acute muscle strain, he may as well forego it in the majority of cases. Acute muscle spasm will recur on the way home, and results will be poor. The same may well be true of a patient requiring rest who must walk long distances or climb stairs to get home from a clinic.

Such cases require hospitalization. If admission to the hospital is not possible, such patients should receive home treatment or be referred to more favorably situated clinics.

PART 2
THE APPLICATION OF THERAPEUTIC EXERCISES TO PARTICULAR FIELDS

Chapter 7

MUSCULO-SKELETAL APPARATUS

INDICATIONS FOR THERAPEUTIC EXERCISES

THE ULTIMATE AIM of orthopedics and traumatology is maximum restoration of function. Exercises* and management of muscle pain are, therefore, integral parts of any treatment plan. After acute trauma, immediate active motion should be started as soon as possible, preferably at once. Besides preserving joint range and muscle strength, active motion will help improve local circulation, reduce intra-- and extra-articular swelling. This, in turn, aids reparative processes such as callus formation.

The muscle plays a vital role in forming the structure of the bones. Function interrelates and frequently precedes form. Exercise is, therefore, essential in the treatment of orthopedic deformity in childhood.

In acute trauma, the final aim of the treatment is frequently to restore full and perfect function. This may depend on restoring perfect structure first; frequently, however, this is a secondary requirement. *Anatomy should be regarded as a basis for function, not as an end in itself.*

---

* It should be recalled that the term (*see* page 7) and dosage of an exercise decides its value. The same movement will have different effects depending on the way it is performed and depending on the case. For example: the exercise "Arms extended at side of body, touch shoulder with fist, return to starting position" can be used for strength building of elbow flexion, increase of elasticity of same (*see* Fig. 3) or it can be used as an exercise for the triceps.

The movements described will therefore be simple. The way they are carried out: against gravity, resistance given, assistance given, dosage etc. will determine the use of the exercise.

Therefore the movements described as examples in the following pages receive a meaning only when considered as *a part of the accompanying paragraphs.*

It is attempted to describe simple movements and only a few of them for every case group. This is especially true for the "extremities." In trunk exercises in which movements are much harder to analyze, more examples are given.

Acute trauma to the bone poses these immediate questions: First is external or internal fixation of the injured part necessary? Secondly, if so, how can immobilization be accomplished most effectively and with minimal restriction of movement?

It is the responsibility of the surgeon to determine when a bone or joint can be exposed to the influence of gravity, weight-bearing, muscle pull, or to the combined influences of more than one of these factors. He will make clear when, in his opinion, an extremity—or part of one—is ready for one or all of these influences. From that point on, the physiotherapist should be able to prepare a program covering type and degree of exercise. This division of responsibility must be kept clear in the minds of all members of the *treatment team;* otherwise, disappointments over results of the procedure will be inevitable.

In the following pages a few surgical approaches are outlined, not as illustrations of what is specifically desired or preferred, but simply to make more real and concrete the examples cited and the problems presented.

The surgeon must decide what form of fixation, if any, is necessary. The physical therapist, interested in obtaining maximum motion as quickly as possible, will prefer the method that gives this mobility. When early motion is made possible (e.g., by internal fixation), the advantage gained should never be lost by delaying active motion. In most cases active motion may be started long before permitting normal use of the injured part.

Immediate mobilization frequently leads to the best results and a few instances should be enumerated:

(1) Fracture of the thoracic and lumbar vertebrae without neurological complication, if these fractures do not comprise the pedicles.

(2) Fracture of the rami pubis of pelvis, if uncomplicated.

(3) Fractures of the acetabulum may need traction or surgery before mobilization, but frequently they respond best to immediate mobilization through exercise. The exercise is done lying, postponing weight-bearing for many months.

(4) Most plateau fractures of the tibia do very well when immediately mobilized, with or without balance suspension.

(5) Fractures of the fibula and fractures of the short bones

of the foot, especially the os calcis, if uncomplicated, as well as of the metatarsals, frequently do better without fixation but with immediate mobilization provided the existing position can be accepted. In the upper extremity, fractures of the head of the humerus and fractures of the phalanges and metacarpals, disability can be shortened by many weeks if they are mobilized instead of splinted.

If bedrest and immobilization is necessary, immediate active motion for all free parts of the affected extremity and a general conditioning regime of exercises are indicated, possible complications of the case permitting.

Exercises should continue and be increased during the surgical period of treatment. There should be no sudden jump, no wide gap, between the period of fixation and the so-called after-treatment period when fixation and support have been dispensed with. After-treatment should continue to strengthen the parts not immediately affected, to mobilize them in so far as their mobility may have been impaired, and to concentrate on the part that has not previously been free for exercise.

Muscle test is the basis for the exercise program. It is understood that examination and diagnosis of the injury proper has preceded the muscle test, and that the diagnosis has first bearing on management. Weak muscles should receive strengthening exercises; foreshortened muscles should be actively and passively lengthened. Active use, and especially weight-bearing, should not be attempted until the extremity is ready.

Co-ordination does not usually create a special problem in the treatment of fractures. Sometimes, however, after strength and elasticity have been restored to their maximum, poor co-ordination may remain, as a result of insufficiency of individual muscles or muscle groups. In the field of skeletal injury, restoring co-ordination is the job of the occupational therapy workshop rather than of special exercises.

The objective in the treatment of fracture is not only to obtain full function, as previously mentioned, but to obtain this *full function in as short a time as possible.* Many fractures eventually get fairly well as a result of almost any proper treatment. Planned exercise therapy should aim to reduce considerably the treatment period and to bring function back to as close to normal as possible. When this goal is unattainable, compensation for function that cannot be restored must be substituted. Treatment should be terminated when no further improvement has been attained for a period of time, or when full function has been attained. Full function means the return, not only to a specific activity, but, if possible, to *all* activities desired or desirable on the part of the patient.

The indication differs for old fractures with residual disabilities, or old orthopedic complaints. Exercises should not be started unless the patient genuinely wants to improve his physical state. The fact must be emphasized that treatment will require a long period of time, and that, out of this, a certain, shorter, period will be needed to find out whether or not improvement is even possible.

The patient must furthermore be informed of all necessary personal restrictions—as to rest, modified working conditions, etc.—and the changes in his personal routine on which depends any measure of success. He will have to understand that his co-operation is essential and that without it treatment will be stopped, because the procedure can then be of no value.

Attention must be given to the attitude of a chronic patient who wants to hand his ailment over to the doctor, expecting effortless relief, or who may not wish relief so much as attention. This mentality can be avoided in most cases of acute trauma when the patient co-operates from the start by active exercise.

In old trauma and in many orthopedic conditions, perfect function is not to be expected. The final purpose of treatment will frequently be more modest: return to any kind of work, return to fairly normal daily routine, return to a tolerable sort of life. Often exercises must be kept up for long periods and may have to be resumed at frequent intervals in order to maintain minimum standards of well-being.

Long duration of exercise treatment applies likewise to orthopedic conditions in the growing years. Posture exercises, for instance, may have to be carried on, or at least resumed at regular intervals, until the end of growth. In children, however, the attitude toward treatment must be much more positive, and both child and parent encouraged rather than discouraged—this being in contrast to adult chronic cases, in which treatment should be discontinued if co-operation is not forthcoming. It is the duty of the consulting physician to stress the importance of exercise therapy as well as its difficulties, and to impress upon the parents their obligation toward the child, in order to make conservative treatment possible.

Before and after bone surgery, exercises should be given to create the best possible circumstances for operation, and to derive the most functional value from that procedure.

In fracture as well as in orthopedic services, group treatment may suggest itself. Frequently individual treatment is not feasible or is only so in special cases. A large number of patients and a small number of therapists make group treatment necessary.

Group treatment has certain advantages and should be considered even when individual attention is available. The awareness of competition has a beneficial effect, so does the feeling of being not isolated or unique in one's disability, and likewise the active and constructive spirit of a well-organized group.

Groups may be formed according to types of disability. They may be graded, again according to relative progression, and the individual given, if necessary, a few additional and special exercises.

Since the function of the *joint* is movement or transmission of movement, immobilization will have particularly serious effects on the joints. Likewise, the constantly repeated incorrect use of any joint will produce functional and structural pathology. This fact is especially obvious in the lower extremities and in the joints of the spine, but is equally to be observed in joints of the upper extremity.

Exercise plays an important part in the treatment of chronic arthritis. As always, pain has to be relieved or at least minimized when motion is started, and as always examination and diagnosis will have to precede the muscle test and have first bearing on management.

When movement is possible, it is again important to evaluate not only the quality of muscle function requiring exercise but the degree of weakness; contracture and spasm should be gauged and as well defined as possible. In the treatment of pain one will do well to palpate for triggerpoints in the muscles, an examination that should be part of any standard appraisal of the musculoscaletal apparatus.

It is important to remember that limitation of motion in a joint will not only depend on contracture of the muscle but contracture of capsule and ligament may be present as well. These fibrous contractures rarely respond to exercises.

In acute trauma or in acute non-infectious conditions, immediate or at least early motion is preferable. Early mobilization does not necessarily mean early use of the extremity especially not early weight bearing.

The use of surface anesthesia is often of great help in therapeutic exercises for bones and joints. Surface anesthetics help raise the pain limit and make amenable to immediate mobilization conditions that might otherwise require long rest periods. The use of surface anesthesia also has its place in the treatment of fractures and chronic orthopedic cases when movement is indicated, yet pain interferes with movement.

The very large group of injuries, commonly classified as *"sprains"* is subject for immediate mobilization with the help of local anesthetics provided major ligament tear or internal injuries of the joint have been excluded.

The treatment of muscle injury—*strain*—is subject to the same considerations. Muscle strain may appear after a fall or other external trauma, or after "internal" trauma produced by fast or unprepared-for movement by which a muscle is pulled by its antagonists, and cannot relax quickly enough to give way to the antagonist's action.

Low temperatures, fatigue, prolonged rest or lack of training seem to increase the chances for strains. Fast movements—running, jumping, vaulting, throwing—and certain every day movements, such as sudden stopping, bending or getting up from a chair, all may produce strain. Lack of warm-up followed by cooling of the affected muscles by draught, or fatigue of these muscles, frequently occur in case histories.

There may or may not be a *pain-free and symptom-free in-*

terval. Relatively severe acute muscle strains often set in without such an interval; minor ones may appear after an interval of sometimes, several hours.

After diagnosis has excluded major tears of muscle or tendon, relief of pain and immediate active motion should be started. Type and degree of motion is always being determined by appraisal of muscle function.

Many acute muscle strains *become chronic*, either by inadequate management or by repeated reinjury.

Residual weakness, stiffness and triggerpoints can be the cause for many years of recurrent pain and disability.

Muscle strains are frequently disregarded. Attention is paid more frequently to bone, joint and ligament than to the muscle as a much too neglected part of the human anatomy.

It is increasingly understood that poor muscle function or muscle injury are at least in part responsible for many orthopedic complaints such as stiff neck, painful shoulders, "osteo arthritic" knees, back pain, etc.

It is desirable to diagnose and treat such complaints with full consideration of the muscular components.

Major trauma to the muscle, major tears or complete tears of tendons, may require surgical treatment or immobilization. In such cases, the non-immobilized part of the extremity should be treated according to principles outlined for bone and joint injuries. As soon as the muscle has been returned to function, the affected groups of muscles should undergo a gradually increasing period of strengthening, and lengthening.

The common problems in acute and chronic muscle strain are: (1) relieving pain during motion, (2) increasing elasticity when impaired and (3) increasing deficient muscle strength. It will not always be possible to achieve all these objectives, especially the last two. Indeed, in chronic cases, compensation may have to be tried for, that is, compensation of a weak muscle by strengthening the synergist or changing the gait or reach or by

---

* Systemic muscle diseases—muscle dystrophy, hypertrophy or pseudo-hypertrophy—will be discussed in connection with lesions of the lower motor neuron lesion.

the use of additional joints and muscles when one or more have been limited by contracture.

In chronic cases the use of deep heat (short wave, diathermy) is helpful in counteracting this shortening and should always be followed by active exercises and by passive stretching, if necessary; passive stretching, in these cases, often causes discomfort. If there is pain after treatment, surface anesthetics may be needed; pain lasting overnight after treatment must be considered a sign of overdosage.

In chronic conditions it is not only necessary to restore elasticity and thereby full range, but frequently certain muscle groups will be found to have lost strength to such a point that they have either to be re-trained carefully or substituted for by others (when possible).

Other assistive measures such as injection of triggerpoints may be necessary in the treatment of these chronic strains. Pinching massage is sometimes required for fibrositis, which may be so marked that it hides triggerpoints at the beginning of treatment.

Patients with chronic muscular deficiencies sometimes offer difficult emotional problems ranging from attention seeking to dependence on indemnities. If the patient shows an undue amount of emotional involvement, physical therapy becomes useless and may only be employed as a facet of overall psychiatric management.

CONTRA-INDICATIONS

Contra-indications for exercises in *the treatment of the musculo-skeletal apparatus* are the presence of tumors in the affected regions, acute and chronic inflammation conditions if not well under control. Exercises are not prescribed if there are complicating conditions of the soft parts and of the skin.

Infections of the joint are another contra-indication. However, exercises are indicated as soon as the basic illness is under control. In such instances, exercises often contribute to preserving or restoring function.

Exercises should not be performed when recent fractures, tears of ligaments, tendons and muscles require surgical repair or external fixation, or when after surgery or immobilization sufficent healing is not yet present. Under all circumstances, the individual case histories must receive careful attention.

Active motion is not identical with full use of an extremity especially not with weight bearing. When graded and appropriate therapeutic exercises may be beneficial, return to uncontrolled use of injured part may retard rehabilitation and even prevent complete restoration of function.

Back

Exercises for backpain and for fractures of the spine are largely based on posture work. The correction of faulty posture should be based on appraisal of structural and functional measurements and requires meticulous work and frequent strictly prescribed exercise sessions, at least two or three times a week, under supervision, followed up by regular home exercises. Instructions of how to stand or walk properly may be a part of the program, but without adequate muscle training they are useless. It is unrealistic to expect success from a few minutes instructions given once a week or even less often. The forces producing poor pos-

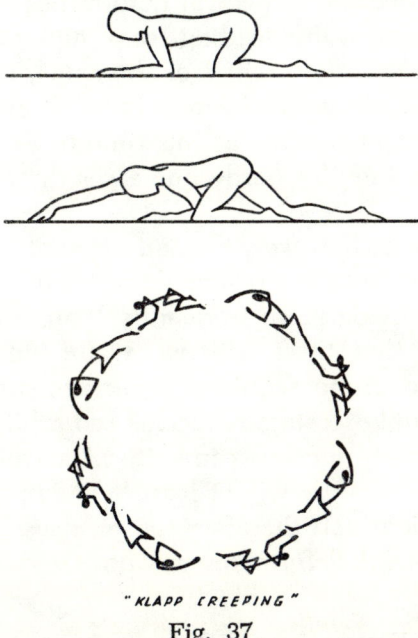

"KLAPP CREEPING"
Fig. 37

ture which include habit, emotional strain, occupation, influence of surroundings and other factors, operate almost incessantly and it is optimistic to expect a few minutes of work to be sufficient to undo these strong and permanent influences. Posture work insufficiently performed will, therefore, yield poor results and it is due to the fact that few patients and unfortunately few therapists find enough time for the necessary effort and regularity that effective posture training is only rarely to be found. Yet, good posture work, besides producing satisfactory results in properly selected cases, is the basis for understanding of therapeutic exercises for chronic and acute back injury.

We shall, therefore, start this section with the description of posture evaluation and posture exercises.

POSTURE*

The large group of mild and moderately severe cases of poor posture require exercise treatment, as well as do the severe cases that need such treatment before or after orthopedic procedure.

It seems likely that some of the more serious cases of "poor posture" finally become structural deformities necessitating surgery. If we visualize a line leading from mild postural anomalies to the graver skeletal deformities of the spine, it will be obvious that exercises will aid in the former, but will not succeed in the severe cases. It is impossible at this time to fix a dividing point on this imaginary line; for borderline cases the criteria are as yet insufficient.

It does appear, however, that an attempt to improve borderline cases, or at least to prevent them from becoming surgical cases, should be made more frequently than is done at present. The assumption that there are two well-defined categories of cases, one a mild group requiring no treatment at all, and the other amenable only to surgery, seems too arbitrary to be valid.

When deformity increases in spite of a well-managed exercise program, the exercise will at least have improved the muscle status of the patient and therefore the prognosis. Exercises after operations for spinal deformities are now widely accepted and

---

* Pictures from KRAUS, HANS and WEBER, S. E.: Evaluation of Posture Based on Structural and Functional Measurements. *Physiol. Rev.* 26:6, 1945.

should be started much sooner than usual. At first, they should follow the exercises described under back pain (p. 132) for fracture of the spine. Only after immobilization has been completely discarded, and free movement has been allowed, should spinal posture training be resumed.

The following measurements are helpful as a basis for such an exercise program:

Structural Measurements

Unless otherwise specified, all measurements are taken from standing position, in the absence of pain. The patient is asked to stand with feet one or two inches apart, the weight of the body being evenly distributed on both feet, with knees straight, looking directly ahead at a mark at eye level on an opposite wall. The body should be relaxed and inactive, the arms hanging at the sides. Let the patient stand in this position for one or two minutes to allow him to sink into habitual alignment, before beginning measurement. Marking the anatomical points on the patient with a skin pencil facilitates measurement.

Chest expansion measurement is taken in inches over the xyphoid bone, (a) in neutral or midway position, (b) on extreme inspiration and (c) on extreme expiration.

Scapulae-spine distance is given in inches and measured from the posterior process of the dorsal vertebra at the level of the inferior medial angle of the scapula, to the inferior medial angle of the same scapula. Measurement is repeated on the other side. A caliper is used to ascertain the distance, which is then read off on a ruler.

Level of the scapulae is measured by placing a water level ruler so that it touches the inferior angle of the scapulae. If the water level shows that they are not horizontal, the water level is held horizontal at the lower scapula and extended across the back beneath the other scapula. A caliper is then used to measure the distance to the higher scapula from the water level held at the lower scapula.

Level of the anterior-superior spine of the ilium is measured by placing the water level at the level of the anterior superior spines of the iliac bones marked by skin pencil. If the water level shows them not to be in horizontal alignment, it is held at the

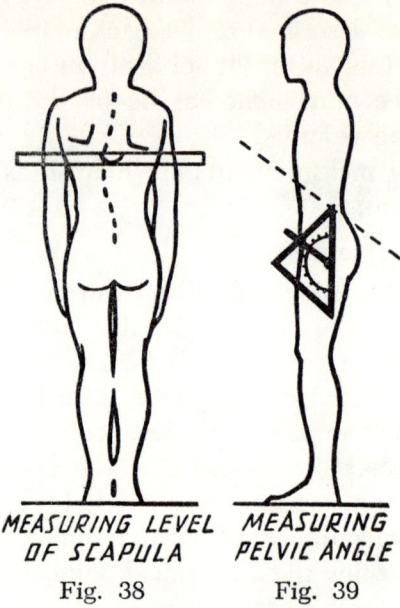

MEASURING LEVEL OF SCAPULA
Fig. 38

MEASURING PELVIC ANGLE
Fig. 39

lower of the two ilia. The distance between water level and the higher ilium is taken with a caliper.

Length of legs is taken with a steel band. The patient should be supine on the table, and the distance from the anterior superior spine of the ilium to the internal malleolus is then measured.

Angle of pelvic tilt is measured with a protractor. The protractor is held against the lateral aspect of the hip joint so that the straight line 0° to 180° is parallel to the long axis of the femur.

Be sure the knee is not bent. The arm of the protractor is then adjusted so that it is parallel to the sacrum. The obtuse angle between the 0°-180° line and the arm of the protractor is read off. The normal reading will be 160°-165° degrees.

Dorsal kyphosis and lumbar lordosis are gauged by taking three measurements. The patient is placed with back to a plumb line suspended from the ceiling. The distances from the plumb line to respectively, (*see* Fig. 40):

    (a) the posterior process of the seventh cervical vertebra,
    (b) the posterior process of the vertebra at the apex of the kyphosis, and

Musculo-Skeletal Apparatus

(c) the posterior process of the fifth lumbar vertebra are measured, using a calibrated water level ruler. The degree of dorsal kyphosis and lumbar lordosis is then computed by taking the apex of the kyphosis as reference 0, and reading and subtracting its distance to the plumb line from the other distances. For example (*see* Fig. 40):

Reading on Ruler	Referred to Apex 0
7 cervical V. 7½ in.	6¼
Apex (kyphotic) 1¼ in.	0
5 lumbar V. 5½ in.	4¼

Functional Measurements

Length of muscles measured by the maximum degree of active joint range indicates muscle elasticity.

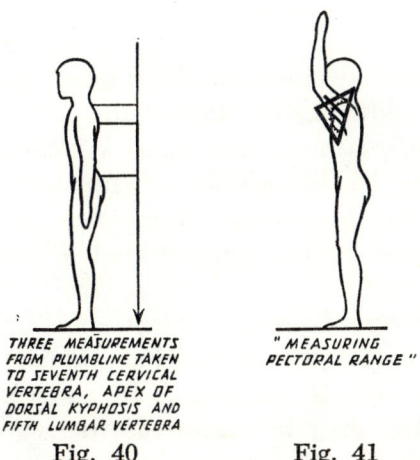

THREE MEASUREMENTS FROM PLUMBLINE TAKEN TO SEVENTH CERVICAL VERTEBRA, APEX OF DORSAL KYPHOSIS AND FIFTH LUMBAR VERTEBRA

Fig. 40

"MEASURING PECTORAL RANGE"

Fig. 41

Total elasticity of the pectoral muscles (Fig. 41) is measured by the angle formed by the arm, when fully raised, with a line parallel to the longitudinal axis of the thorax. The patient is asked to raise one arm as high as possible in a forward direction, pointing toward the ceiling. Then the protractor is held laterally against the shoulder joint, with the straight of 0°-180° parallel to the longitudinal axis of the thorax. The arm of the protractor is adjusted parallel to the lengthwise axis of the humerus, and the obtuse angle is read off. This is repeated on the opposite side. The normal muscle will give a reading of 170° to 180°.

Total Elasticity of Hamstrings is measured by the angle to which one leg of patient can be lifted passively with knee straight. Normal is about 80°.

Total elasticity of the hamstring and gluteal muscles is measured by the angle to which the legs may be lifted from a supine position without causing motion in the lumbar of the spine. To take this measurement the patient must be completely relaxed in supine position on the table. The protractor is placed with the straight line of 0°-180° on the treatment table next to the patient's hip joint. The examiner places his fingers lightly on the posterior spinal processes of the 4th and 5th lumbar vertebrae, sliding his hand gently under the patient's back. An assistant slowly lifts both legs, holding them by ankles or heels. The patient must remain completely relaxed throughout the test. The instant the examiner feels motion in the lumbar spine, the full length of the hamstrings has been reached, and a further lifting of the legs causes movement of the lumbar vertebrae in a posterior direction. When this motion in the lumbar spine is felt by the examiner, the assistant stops the slow lifting motion and hold the legs at this angle. The arm of the protractor is then adjusted parallel to the lengthwise axis of the femur and the acute angle between table level and the femur is read off the protractor. Normal about 35°.

Total elasticity of erector spinae and hamstring muscles: The patient is asked to bend forward and touch the floor with the fingertips of both hands. Care must be taken that the knees remain straight. The distance from the fingertips to the floor is measured with a ruler. Normally proportioned individuals will be able to touch fingertips to the floor.

Muscle Strength and Holding Power Measurements

(a) *"Lower abdominal" strength.* The patient lies on his back, lifting both legs to an angle of 30° and holding this position unassisted, with his hands behind head. Ability to maintain the position for ten seconds is considered an indication of normal

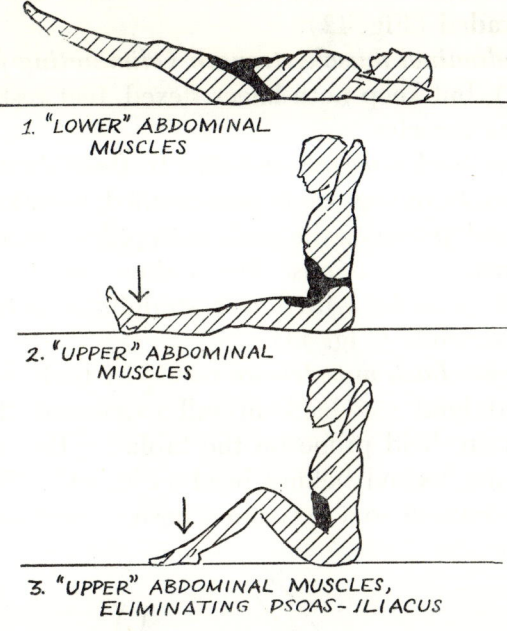

Fig. 42

holding power (Fig. 42).

(b) *"Upper abdominal" strength:* The patient lies in a supine position, hands clasped behind neck. If he is able to raise his trunk from this position to 90° without assistance, his "upper

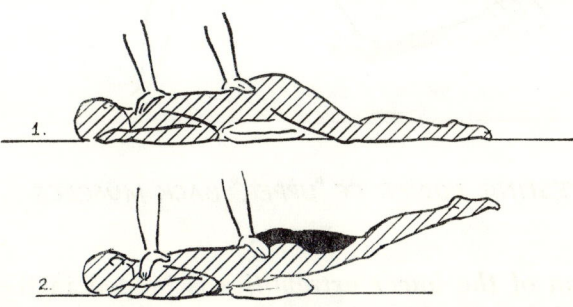

Fig. 43

abdominal" power is counted as 100% (10). If help is needed up to a 45° angle is considered 50% (5), and subdivisions are correspondingly graded (Fig. 42).

(c) *Abdominal muscle strength* (*eliminating psoasiliacus*). Test as in (b), but keep both knees flexed, feet resting on table.

Erector spinae muscles

(a) *Lower back muscles* are tested by their ability to stabilize the pelvis when both legs are hyperextended, with knees straight. Patient has trunk prone on the table with pillow under hips, holds on to table with both hands. He is then asked to extend his hips as far as possible, with knees straight, and to hold them there for ten seconds (Fig. 43).

(b) *Upper back muscles* are tested by their ability to raise the trunk and hold the back in full extension. The patient's legs and hips are held prone on the table by the examiner. Patient's hands are locked behind head (Fig. 44). The patient is asked to raise himself to a horizontal position and hold it for ten seconds.

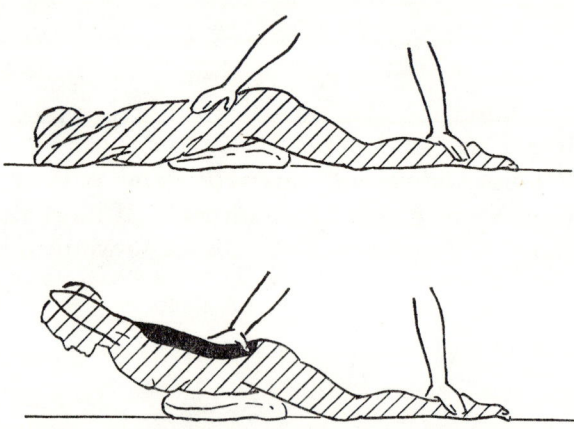

TESTING POWER OF "UPPER" BACK MUSCLES

Fig. 44

Position of the lower extremities is judged in the standard position and described by the usual nomenclature; inversion and eversion at the hip, genu valgum or recurvatum at the knee, and pronation or supination of feet particularly.

Breathing is observed in supine and in erect position and marked as: (a) abdominal, (b) predominant abdominal, (c) chest, (d) predominant chest, and (s) abdominal and chest equally.

INTERPRETATION OF MEASUREMENTS

To interpret the measurements one must always keep in mind the individual case as a whole. Should any structural deformity be present, it must be noted on the measurement record. In such instances, the measurements give supplementary data to the x-ray report. Disregarding such cases of abnormal bony structure, the following interpretation will fit the general run of posture cases:

INTERPRETATION OF STRUCTURAL MEASUREMENTS

The chest expansion measurement is of value in determining relative expansion and breathing capacity.

The measurements of the scapulae-spine distances, if unequal, may help gauge the lateral curve of the dorsal spine, the apex on the side of the smaller scapula-spine distance. This is possible if asymmetries of the shoulder girdle are taken into consideration as well as their level and the level of the anterior-superior spines of the pelvis and the clinical aspect.

The use of a water level to determine the level of the scapulae is obvious. The presence of an uneven level may be associated with a lateral curve of the spine or a disturbance in the distribution of tension in the muscles of the shoulder girdle.

The level of the anterior-superior spine of the ilium, if not horizontal, indicates a lateral tilt of the pelvis. This may be interpreted as possibly correlated with a scoliosis in the lumbar spine with the apex to the side of the lower ilium.

If the measurements show that one leg is shorter than the other, it is usual to associate corresponding lateral tilt of the pelvis and a curvature in the lumbar spine with the apex of the curve to the side of the shorter leg. This is a direct result of short-leg function.

The measurements of the angle of the forward pelvic tilt

showing figures lower than 160° indicate an increased lumbar lordosis, whereas figures higher than 170° indicate flat backs.

The measurements for dorsal kyphosis and lumbar lordosis show an increase of the curves in direct proportion to the increase in distance between the 7th cervical and 5th lumbar vertebrae, to the apex of the curve marked 0°, and a corresponding decrease if these distances have decreased.

INTERPRETATION OF FUNCTIONAL MEASUREMENTS

Muscle Length and Elasticity

Pectoralis muscles: An angle of less than 170° to 180° indicates a shortened pectoralis muscle group, which is usually associated with an anterior displacement of the shoulder, a narrow chest, restricted range of movement in the shoulder joint, and possible dorsal kyphosis.

Hamstrings: Are foreshortened if single leg raise is less than 80°.

Gluteal and hamstring muscles: If the angle measured is less than 35° a shortness of the hamstring and gluteal muscle groups is indicated.

Erector spinae, gluteal and hamstring muscles: In the bending test, the distance from fingertips to the floor gives an indication of the length of both back and hamstring muscles. Comparison of this test with the one above indicates whether the erector spinae, gluteal, or hamstring muscles or all these muscle groups are contractured.

Muscle Strength and Holding Power

In these measurements, muscle strength is tested according to its ability to overcome gravity by assuming the test position. The holding power of the muscle is measured by the time the patient can hold the position.

Position of the lower extremities and the patient's breathing are observed and described. Consideration must always be given to the fact that tendencies to abdominal and chest breathing vary at different ages in children. In adolescents and adults the type of breathing also varies according to sex.

Posture Exercises

Exercises are prescribed according to the deficiencies found through the above measurements. The following exercises, which are some that may be used in the treatment of poor posture, should be regarded as examples rather than as definite recommendations, but they have proved satisfactory in both group and individual treatment.

Most of the severe cases should receive individual treatment, and it is obvious that all exercises should be adapted to the particular patient. Frequently individual and group treatment can be combined by warming up the patient in a group and then giving individual exercises for his special requirements.

Exercises are graded: A-mild, B-moderate, and C-strenuous. This grading is used (1) to build up the exercise program, and (2) as a warm-up for each single session, which starts with mild exercises, works up to medium and strenuous ones and then returns to mild exercises as a "cool-off."

Breathing Exercises

(A) *Double Breathing:* Patient lying on back, hands locked behind head, knees flexed. Breath in through nose, raising ribs (relaxed shoulders). Breath out through mouth, lowering ribs as far as possible, making a hissing sound.

(A) *"Single Breathing":* Give patient mental picture of each lung (red and blue balloon). Patient lying on back, hands locked behind head, knees flexed, shoulders relaxed. Breath in through nose, concentrating on one side, stretching shoulder and elbow up. Exhale, moving shoulder and elbow down again. Press all air out, lowering ribs as far as possible, making a hissing sound. Relax. Repeat on other side.

(A) *Breathing with Lateral Arm Swing:* Patient lying on back, arms at side of body, knees flexed. Swing arms over head and sideways, breathing in through nose—stretch—breath out through mouth—hissing—swinging arms down. Relax.

(A) *Breathing with Forward Arm Swing:* Same as 3, but swinging arms forward and overhead.

(A) *Prone Breathing:* Patient lying prone, head resting on folded arms. Breath in through nose, breath out through mouth with hissing sound, physical threapist helping to exhale and lower ribs. Relax.

(A) *One-Sided Breathing in Lateral Position:* Patient lying on his right or left side over hard flat pillow placed under ribs. Right or left arm with bent elbow over head. Breath in through nose, breath out—hissing—through mouth. Relax (Fig. 86).

(B) *Standing Breathing:* Patient standing leans forward, arms dangling. Stretch arms over head, rising to erect position on toes, breathing in. Drop forward, breathing out through mouth, hissing. Relax. Repeat (Fig. 87).

(A) *Abdominal Breathing:* Patient on back, arms at sides, knees flexed. Breath in and out, raising and lowering abdomen, with or without resisting weight on abdomen.

(B) *Chest and Abdominal Breathing:* Position as in 8: Breath in through nose, expanding first abdomen, then chest. Breath out through mouth, hissing, lowering first abdomen, then chest.

Stretch of Gastrocnemius Soleus

(A) *Standing Double Stretch*: Patient stands about two feet from table, hands placed on table, leaning forward, bending elbows, keeping hip and knee joints straight, heels pressed to floor. Stretch elbows and stand erect. Relax.

(B) *Standing Single Stretch Soleus:* Patient stands with right or left foot forward, places hands on right or left knee, then leans forward, flexing right or left knee, pressing downward with both hands. Return to erect position. Relax.

Abdominal Exercises

(A) *Tip-Up:* Patient lying on back, hands locked behind head, knees bent. Patient pulls abdomen up and in, slightly raising buttocks and pressing lumbar spine against table (Fig. 45).

(A) *Flexion and Extension:* Patient lying on back. Flex right leg and left arm so that knee and elbow touch, then stretch to full extension. Flex left leg and right arm so that knee and elbow touch, then stretch to full extension. Flex both legs and arms so that right knee-right elbow and left knee-left elbow touch; stretch both legs and arms to full extension. Repeat rhythmically. Relax.

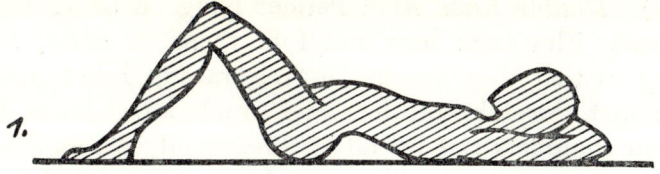

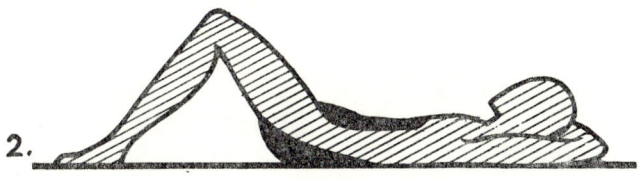

TIPUP
Fig. 45

(A) **Stomach Balloon:** Patient lying on back, hands locked behind head. Patient rises abdomen against resisting hand or sandbag—lowers. Repeat. Relax.

(A) **Abdominal Bridge:** Patient lying face down. Pull abdomen up and in, clearing table. Relax.

(B) **Sitting Up:** Patient lying on back, knees flexed, hands locked, stretched to full extension or held behind head, head and shoulders either on or off table (therapist holds patient's ankles). Patient comes up to sitting position, then gently rolls down to lying position. Relax. Grading can be done by (a) keeping arms at the side of patient, later folded across chest, (b) starting to sit up from an angle of about 45° and lessening the angle until the "sit-up" is done from a horizontal position, or (c) by manual assistance.

(B) **Single Knee Kiss:** Patient lying on back, head and shoulders flat on table throughout exercise. Flex right or left knee and bring thigh up to chest as far as possible (hip and knee in full flexion). Stretch leg to full extension and lower slowly. Repeat on other side. Relax. Graded by starting patient lying on his side.

(A) **Double Knee Kiss:** Patient lying on back, hands behind head. Flex both legs and fold them on chest, bringing them up so that they touch the face, raising lower back from table or mat. Stretch both legs and slowly lower them, holding head and shoulders flat on table throughout exercise. Grading done by starting patient with hip and knees flexed and feet close to buttocks and by gradually increasing distance between buttocks and feet (Fig. 46).

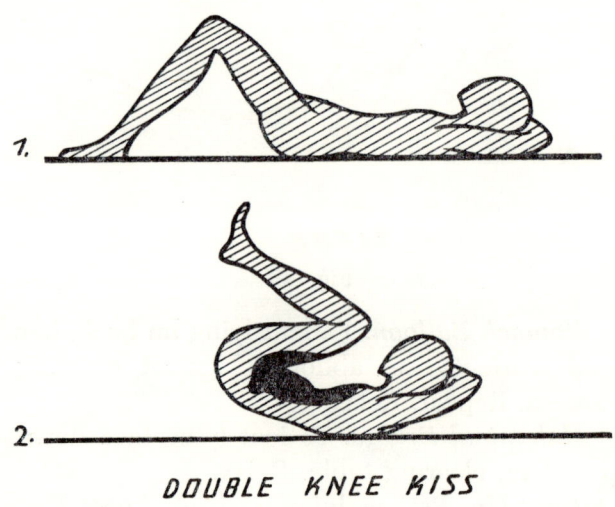

DOUBLE KNEE KISS

Fig. 46

(C) **Leg Circles:** Patient lying flat on table, hands locked behind head. Raise one leg with straight stiff knee to about 45°, describe circle, up to 10 circles. Relax. Repeat with other leg. Relax. Then raise both legs, describe circles up to 10 in both directions. Relax.

(C) **Leg Hold:** Patient lying on back, hands locked behind head. Raise both legs with stiff knees to about 45°. Hold, count to 10. Relax.

(C) **Trunk Swing:** Patient lying on back, hands locked behind head, pelvis fixed (hold pelvis). Raise slightly and swing trunk to left, swing back. Relax. Raise, swing to right, swing back. Relax.

Exercises for Upper Trunk and Shoulder Girdle

(A) *Lying on Sandbag:* Hands locked behind head, knees raised, sandbag placed under shoulders. Patient presses elbows down, tries to touch table. Relax.

(A) *Arm Rotation:* Lying flat on back, arms straight out at sides. Rotate arms backward so that palms face upward. Relax. If done on narrow treatment table, hold elbows flexed so that rotation of upper arm is easily observed.

(A) *Shoulder Circles:* Patient sitting, fingertips on shoulders. Describe circles with elbows starting at side positions, describing circles backwards. Relax after 5-10 circles.

(A) *Sandbag Drop* (Pectoral Stretch): Patient lying on back, arms over edge of table. Saddle sandbag hung over arm in supination.

(B) *Sandbag Lift:* Patient prone on table, arms over edge of table. Patient lifts saddle sandbags to horizontal. Grading by weight of bags.

(B) *Wing Spread:* Patient in sitting position, hands locked behind head or arm straight out at side in horizontal position, palms up. Press arms backwards against resistance. Relax.

(B) *Push-Up:* Patient sitting on table, elbows flexed, palms up. Press palms of therapist upwards until arms are stretched fully at 45° angle upon resistance.

(B) *Arm Spread:* Patient sitting or standing, arms forward, straight elbows: Patient moves arms outward at horizontal against therapist's resistance.

(B) *Turn Door Knob:* (Serratus): Patient sitting or standing. Patient brings arms forward and holds hands of therapist, rotating upper arm outward and hands in supination against therapist's resistance.

(B) *Scapula Pull:* Patient lying prone at edge of table, arm hanging relaxed over edge. Patient pulls shoulder blade toward spine with arm remaining relaxed (Fig. 47).

(B) *Kneeling Back Pull:* Patient on knees, sitting back on heels, hands locked behind back. Drop head forward relaxing back and neck. Then shape back by pulling shoulders backward. Raise head, keep chin in and pull arms downward. Remain in

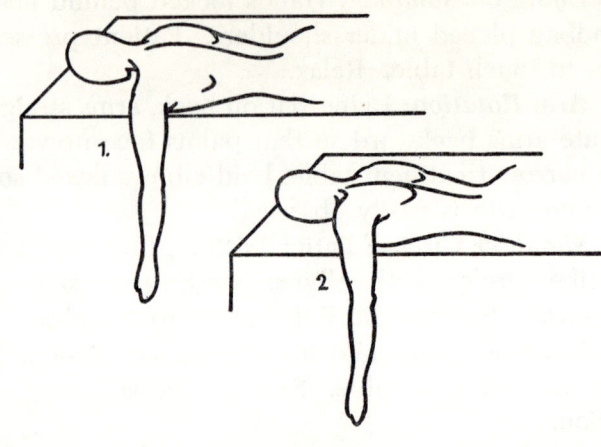

Fig. 47

horizontal position or raise trunk to vertical position (depending on lumbar lordosis or flat back).

(C) *Trunk Raise:* Patient lying on face with head and shoulders on or off table, hands locked behind head. Raise head and upper trunk, pressing shoulders and elbows back, Keep chin in. Relax. Use pillow under hips.

(C) *Aeroplane:* Patient lying face down, head and shoulders on or off table, arms straight out at sides. Raise head and upper trunk, chin in. Turn arms out so that palms face upwards. Relax. Use pillow under hips.

(C) *Rocking Horse:* Patient face down on mat. Take hold of right foot with right hand. Take hold of left foor with left hand. Roll up and rock, chin in. Relax (*see* Fig. 48).

Exercises for Back Mobility and Rotation

(A) *Back Rotation and Flexion:* (a) Patient sitting, legs straight out and slightly apart. Touch right leg or foot with left hand or elbow; touch left leg or foot with right hand or elbow. Relax.

(b) Same as above, but keeping hands locked behind head and turning to each side as far as possible.

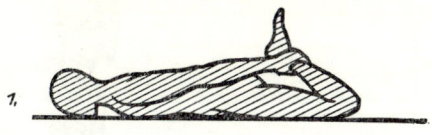
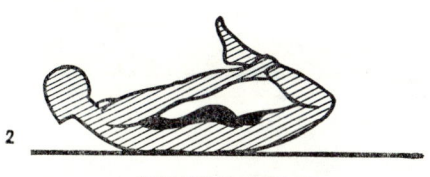

ROCKING HORSE
Fig. 48

(B) **Wind Mill:** Patient standing, legs apart. Swing left arm in a large circle overhead and down, touching back or right foot with fingertips; swing right arm in a large circle overhead, touching left foot with fingertips of right hand. Repeat rhythmically. Relax.

(C) **Leg Kick Over Head:** Patient lying flat on floor, hands locked behind head. Swing both legs over head until toes touch the floor. Legs must be held straight and stiff and together. Swing back, slowly lowering legs to floor. Relax.

(C) **Leg Swing over toward Hand:** Patient lying on floor, flat on back, arms stretched out at sides of body. Touch right hand with left foot, swing leg up and over and back. Touch left hand with right foot. Relax.

Exercises for Hamstring Stretch and Back Mobility

(A) **Toe Touch:** Patient sitting on floor or table, feet against the wall, knees stiff. Touch toes with finger tips. Patient with dorsal kyphosis should keep hands locked behind head, looking up and merely try to bend as far as possible (Fig. 49).

(A) **Standing Bend Over:** Patient standing with straight knees, bends forward, touches toes with fingertips. If kyphosis is present, have patient lock hands behind head and bend body forward, or have hands locked behind back with straight elbows (Fig. 61).

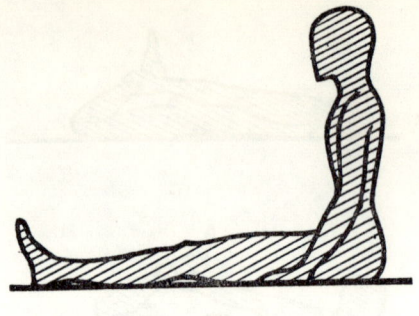

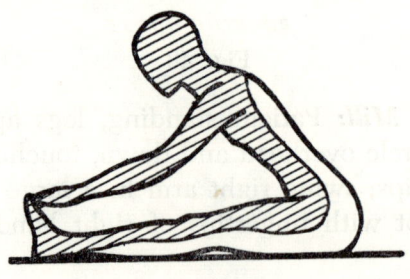

TOE TOUCH

Fig. 49

(A) *Standing Stretch:* Patient standing about two feet from table, holding sides of table with hands. Patient leans forward until body is in horizontal line from hips to head.

(B) *Hamstring Stretch:* Patient lying on back. Take hold of right foot with right hand; stretch knee to full extension. Relax. Hold left foot with left hand, extend knee. Relax. Hold left foot-left hand, right foot-right hand. Extend both knees. Relax.

Neck Exercises

(A) *Accordion:* Lying flat on back, knees flexed, arms relaxed at side. Pull chin down and slide back of head up. Relax. (Fig. 50).

(A) *Forward Flexion:* Assume accordion position, lying flat on back. Raise head from table, touch chest with chin. Relax.

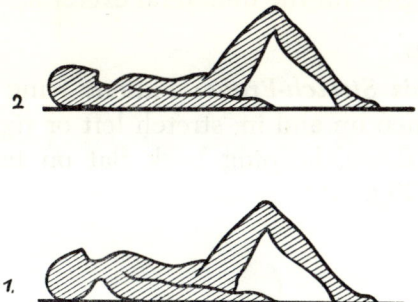

ACCORDION

Fig. 50

(B) *Lateral Flexion:* Assume accordion position, lying flat on back. Raise head ½-in. from table. Bend to right side, bringing ear to shoulder. Return. Relax. Repeat to left side. Relax.

(B) *Rotation:* Assume accordion position. Turn neck toward right. Return. Relax. Turn neck toward left. Return. Relax.

(B) *Sandbag Balance:* Stretch back of head upward, chin pulled in. Balance sandbag on head, walking or running.

(B) *Wall Stretch:* Stand against wall, back and shoulders touching wall. Slide back of head upward, pulling chin in. Relax.

UNILATERAL EXERCISES

In the treatment of scoliosis, regularly repeated back x-rays and orthopedic evaluation are essential. Exercises will, of course, not reverse existing deformity but seem to be able to slow down the rate at which the deformity increases. This is true only if the number of treatment sessions per week is frequent enough (at least 2-3) and if there is good follow-up at home. Cosmetic improvement may be present even if structural changes to the better do not occur, and flexibility of the spine and strength of trunk muscles may be improved to the point where surgery can be more effective. As follow-up after fusion for scoliosis adequate exercise therapy is a MUST to obtain optimum results.

Careful evaluation and muscle test are essential to determine

118 Therapeutic Exercise

the side (left or right) for the unilateral exercise.

Scoliosis Exercises

(A) *Scoliosis Stretch-Prone:* Patient lying face down on table. Pull abdomen up and in, stretch left or right arm up, and left or right leg down, keeping back flat on table throughout exercise. Relax (Fig. 51).

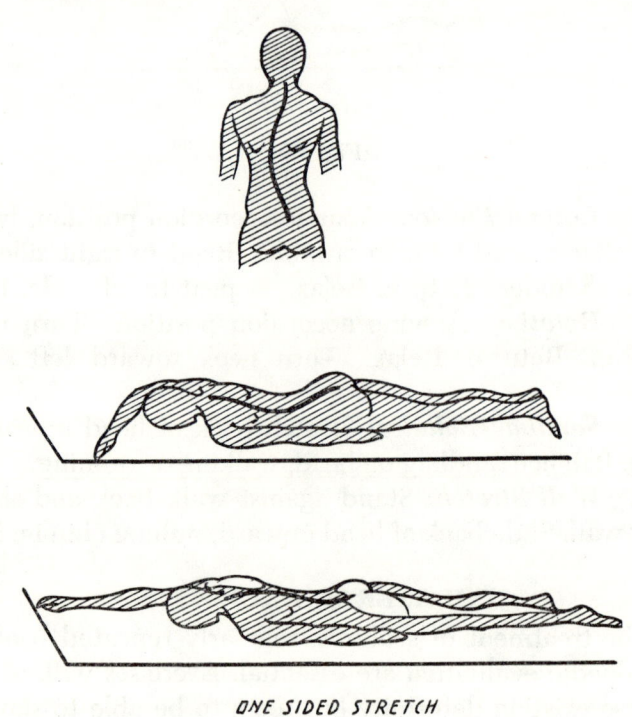

ONE SIDED STRETCH
Fig. 51

(A) *Scoliosis Stretch-Supine:* Patient lying on back, arms at side of body. Stretch left or right arm up, and left or right leg down, keeping back flat on table throughout exercise. Relax.

(A) *Shift:* Patient sitting on table, legs dangling: keep pelvis fixed, lock hands behind head. Stretch spine up, shift upper trunk towards right or left. Keep shoulders horizontal, shift back. Relax (Fig. 52).

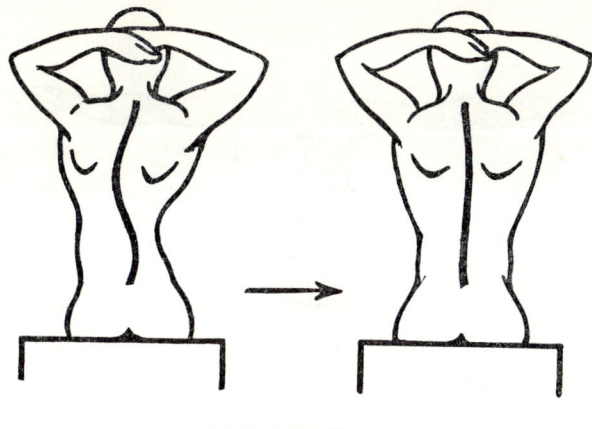

SHIFT
Fig. 52

(A) **One-Sided Shoulder Pull:** Patient sitting with legs over edge of table, arm straight out to side at horizontal, palm up. Pull right or left shoulder blade toward center. Repeat. Relex (Fig. 53).

(B) **Look Up—Look Back:** Patient sitting on table, legs dangling over edge. Lock hands behind head, turn to left or right, raise right or left side (look back and up). Turn back to starting position. Relax.

(B) **Sitting Arm Stretch:** Patient sitting on stool, left or right hand on hip. Stretch right or left arm up in large swinging motion; lower. Relax.

(B) **Shoulder Pull-Up and Hold-Up:** Patient lying or sittting. Therapist holds right or left upper arm and gives resistance while patient raises right or left shoulder. Patient raises right of left shoulder while therapist pulls arm down.

(B) **Lateral Arm Raise:** Patient lying or sitting, raises arm laterally against resistance.

(B) **Turn Door Knob:** (Serratus): Patient sitting or standing, right or left forward. Patient holds hand of therapist and rotates upper arm outward and hand to supination against resistance.

(B) **One-Sided Stretch on Table:** Patient lying face down;

120   *Therapeutic Exercise*

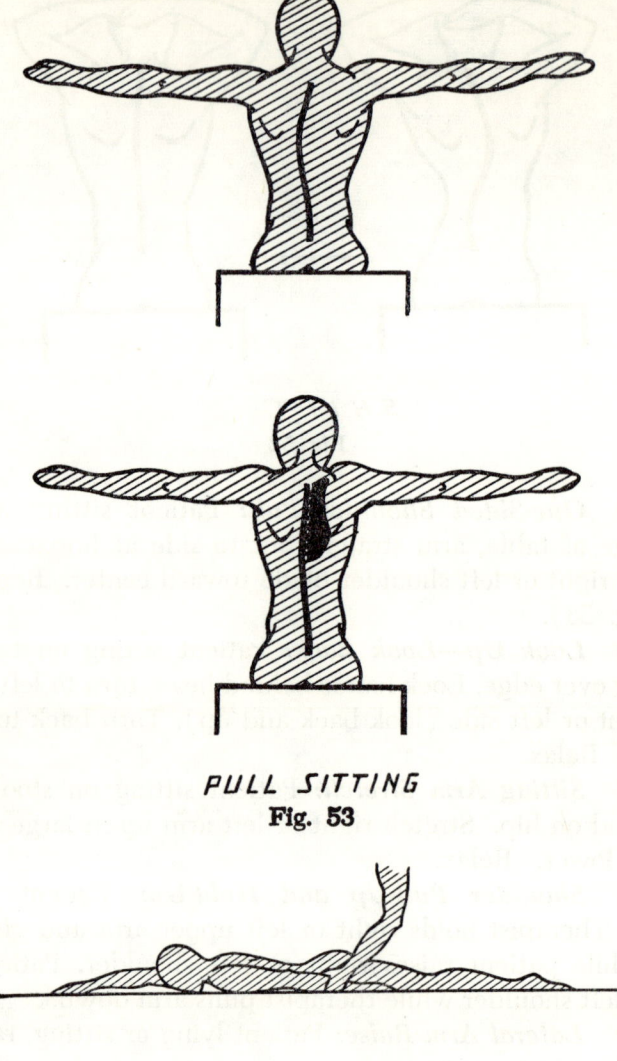

PULL SITTING
Fig. 53

RIGHT-SIDED STRETCH, PRONE
Fig. 54

therapist holds left or right hand in supination and pulls down while patient describes swinging motion with right or left arm, stretching up and raising head and shoulders off table. Swing arm back. (Fig. 54).

(B)   *One-Sided Stretch on Stool:* Patient sits on left or right buttock, stretches right arm and leg, to right, to full extension, or right arm and left leg, or left arm and left leg, or left arm and right leg, leaning body slightly forward. Elbow and knee of extended limb should be in full extension. Return to normal sitting position and relax.

(B)   *Statue:* Patient standing, hands locked behind head. Drop left or right hip by flexing knee, stretch left or right elbow and shoulder upward. Return to normal standing position. Relax.

(C)   *Psoas-iliacus Strength Building:* Patient prone on table, holding sides of table legs, hanging over edge of foot end of table. Therapist holds both legs and supports them at table

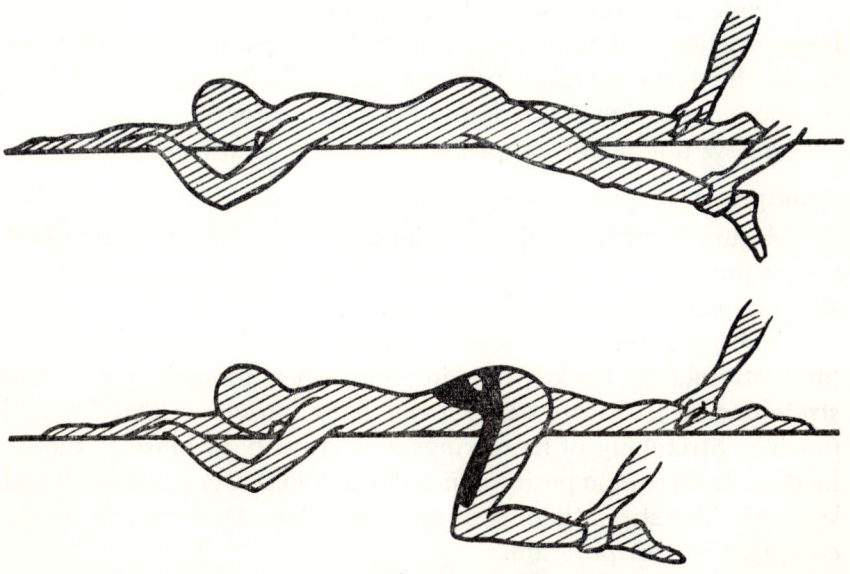

UNILATERAL RESISTANCE TO PSOAS-ILIACUS
(PRONE POSITION PERMITS WATCHING OF SPINE)

Fig. 55

level (horizontal). Patient flexes right or left hip and knee against resistance given by therapist. Relaxes in stretched position. Repeat (Fig. 55).

(C) Same position as above but patient holds right or left leg flexed at hip and knee against pull given by therapist (Holding Power).

(C) *Hip Extension:* Patient prone on table, raises right or left leg with stiff knee against therapist's resistance.

(C) Same position as above: Patient holds right or left leg up with stiff knee (in hip extension) against downward pull exerted by therapist.

Foot Exercises (*see* pages 172-176)

Unilateral exercises should be stressed in most cases of scoliosis and are particularly important in the more severe ones which often show unilateral weakness of the trunk muscles. This condition should be tested for, and, if necessary, special emphasis should be placed on unilateral trunk muscle stretching.

Bilateral exercises cannot be expected to correct deformities, because once unilateral weakness and shortening of muscles has set in, bilateral exercises will automatically be performed in a manner conductive to this functional asymmetry.

A few practical examples are outlined below as guides:

Example A

Assume that the major deficiencies shown on a posture chart are: round back, weak upper and lowed abdominals, short hamstrings, pectorals and back muscles.

The program would omit unilateral exercises and stress pectoral stretching, back stretching of upper thoracic spine and stretching of hamstrings and lower back muscles—all active and passive. Stretching of hamstrings and lower back muscles should be done from supine position in order to avoid accentuating dorsal kyphosis. The strengthening of upper and lower abdominals would complement this program.

Depending on the individual case, the program may start with 15 minutes and work up to 30 minutes, six times a week. Progressive grading of exercises between A and C should be done as quickly as tolerable to the patient.

Example B

Assume scoliosis with apex to the mid-thoracic region on the left, the left scapula lower than the right, and trunk muscles weaker on the left side.

Unilateral exercises would constitute the main part of the program and possibly the only part. Unilateral breathing (left side down, right arm up), unilateral stretching supine (again with right arm up), and sitting and standing with the right arm up, should be stressed. Strength-building exercises for the left trunk muscles and psoasiliacus should be prescribed (Fig. 55).

Example C

Assume all normal posture measurements, but a habit of keeping one shoulder higher than the other, standing with abdomen protruding and in a stooped position.

This case will receive habit-forming exercises and posture instruction rather than any specific posture exercises. The program may be successfully supplemented by general exercises and training in body awareness and management.

The supplementary prescription is particularly important in posture treatment. Sleeping habits (hard mattress, pillow conforming to the width of the shoulders), working habits (relative size of desks and chairs), reading and eyesight, habits of load-carrying in one or the other hand, athletic activities—all must be carefully watched.

Sometimes attitudes in daily life are definitely posture-forming: witness the tightness of the trapezius and pectoral muscles and subsequent round back produced by an apprehensive attitude in a timid child. Posture training without accompanying attention to the cause of the habit will frequently fail. Another cause of poor posture, often observed in adolescent girls with premature development, is the attempt to conceal their bosom in order not to differ from others of their age: short pectorals and a tendency to round back are common consequences. Still another voluntary basis for poor posture is the attitude assumed by young girls of leaning back from the hips, balancing their weight behind the hip joint, to imitate the artificial gait of fashion models.

BACK PAIN

Under this common classification a great number of widely different cases have been lumped together. Low back pain does not, of course, constitute a diagnosis, but only states one of leading symptoms—pain in a certain region of the body. Upon diagnosis, well-defined groups of cases can be differentiated.

Over 80 per cent of back pain is due to muscle deficiency and muscle pain. Our sedentary lives deprive us of exercise necessary to maintain adequate muscular fitness. Constant sitting shortens our back and hamstring muscles and weakens our trunk muscles. We may get along quite well with this minimum of muscular equipment until a trivial occurrence forces us to exceed the present muscle capacity. Then lifting of a light weight, stooping for a period of time, twisting or bending too suddenly may produce an acute muscle strain. This strain may improve with pallitative therapy but leaves the muscles still further weakened and stiffened. Repeated episodes gradually lead to chronic back pain frequently simulating more serious affliction. If chronic back suffering ties in with emotional instability and with repeated outside irritations, it finally becomes a well established illness affecting the physical as well as emotional well being of the patient.

When taking the case history, one should look for different types of pain.

(1) Pain after rest ("jelling pain"), improving after mild activity. (2) Pain after work or connected with work. (3) Pain after standing. (Fatigue Pain). (4) Pain increased by emotional tension or outside irritations. (5) Acute episodes of pain resulting in disabling muscle spasm.

Examination of these patients will at first exclude any serious pathology such as tumors, tuberculosis, ruptures and protrusions of intervertebral discs producing definite neurological symptoms, structurally unstable backs, fractures, osteoporosis, rheumatoid arthritis and others. Only in absence of major pathology can we make the diagnosis of "muscular deficient" back. Often however, definite pathology is associated with muscular weakness and stiffness. In such instances reconditioning of the muscles by systematic exercises and relieving of muscular pain may form an important part of the management of the patient. This is especially true of structurally unstable backs and dics lesions. Rheumatoid arthritis (Marie Struempel) where therapeutic exercises have a large place in conservative management and after surgery. Osteo arthritic changes are frequently found in patients with back pain but do not seem to correlate with the amount of pain experienced. They may often be regarded as incidental findings.

Uncomplicated fractures of the spine if not comprising the articular processes can be managed more often than not by immediate mobilization. *Standard examination of the low back patient is incomplete without thorough appraisal of strength and flexibility of key posture muscles and without palpation of soft parts.*

When possible we are using complete posture evaluation as previously described. In a clinic where large numbers of patients have to be examined, we find strength test for trunk muscles and back muscles and flexibility test for back and hamstring muscles sufficient for a quick appraisal. Gauging of tension **should not be neglected.**

The six basic tests (**Kraus-Weber tests for minimum muscular fitness**) (Fig. 56) are self correlating, that is they test the strength of the patient's muscles against his own weight and flexibility of his back and hamstring muscles against his size. They, therefore, apply to every age, sex and height. These tests have been described in the previous section being part of the postural test but are repeated down below for convenience.

Position: Lying supine, hands behind neck. Examiner holds feet down on table. *Command:* "Keep hands behind neck, roll up into sitting position."

Position: Lying supine, hands behind neck and knees bent. Examiner holds feet down on table. *Command*: "Keep hands behind neck and roll up into sitting position."

Position: Supine, with hands behind neck and legs extended. *Command:* "Keep your knees straight and lift feet ten inches off the table for ten seconds"

Position: Lying prone, with pillow under abdomen, hands behind neck. Examiner holds feet and hips down. *Command:* "Raise trunk and hold for ten seconds."

Position: Prone over pillow. Examiner holds back and hips. *Command:* "Lift legs up, hold for ten seconds."

Position: Standing erect in stockings or bare feet, hands at

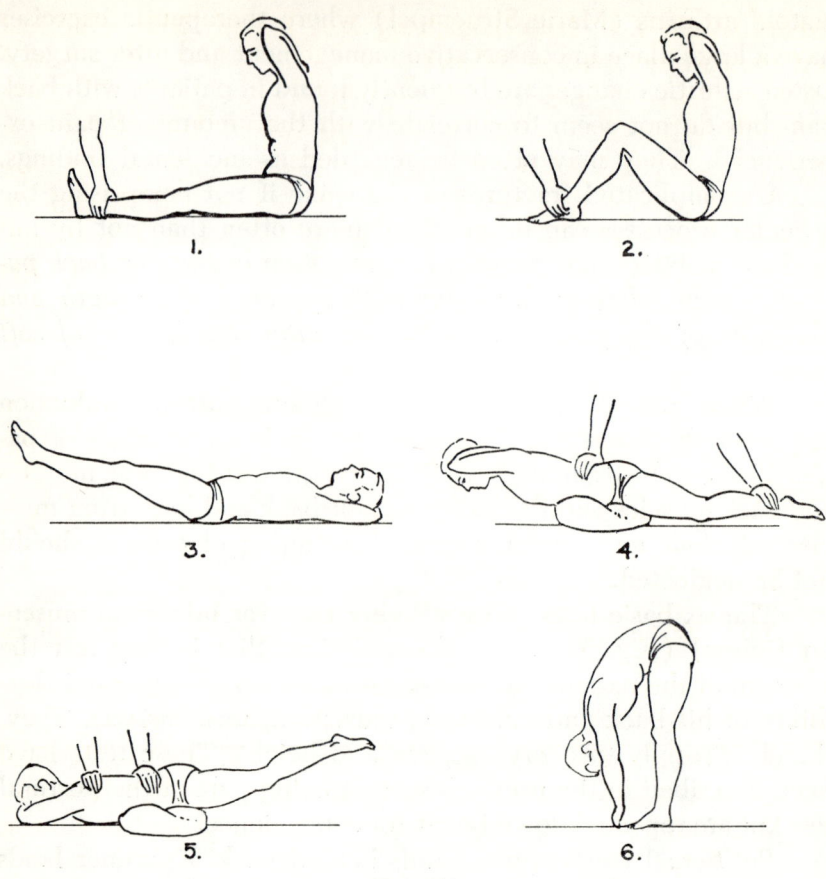

Fig. 56

sides. *Command:* "Put your feet together, keep knees straight, lean down slowly, see how close you can come to touching the floor with your finger tips."

In addition to these basic tests it is helpful to test length of hamstring muscles (passive single leg raise supine).

Palpation of muscles should extend over the whole back and neck and palpation of the skin for fibrositis as well as deep palpation for generalized and localized tenderness (triggerpoints) should be carefully made. (Palpating for triggerpoints, palpating for fibrositis). It is helpful to record results of these tests by indicating abdominal muscle strength by A, back muscle strength with a B, back/hamstring length with BH. A normal test then would read as follows:

$$A \ \frac{10}{10} \ 10 \qquad B\frac{10}{10} \qquad BHT \ (Touch)$$

Figures above the line will stand for "upper back" and "upper abdominal strength", figures below the lower back and lower abdominals (psoas). The third figure for the abdominals will indicate the straigth abdominal strength with psoas elminated. BH indicates hamstring length. In a patient with muscle weakness and stiffness, the test may read:

$$A \ \frac{2}{4} \ 2 \qquad B\frac{8}{9} \qquad BH - 4 \ in.$$

H meaning the hamstring length may be 70 degrees left and 40 degrees right indicating that right hamstrings have been particularly shortened, possibly by repeated episodes of pain in that leg.

These tests should not be performed if there is acute pain.

The exercise program is built on these findings. Examples follow:

Strengthening Exercises for Abdominal Muscles (Graded)
1. "Pelvic tilt." Supine, knees flexed. Tighten abdominal and gluteal muscles to bring small of back to table.
2. Supine, knees flexed. Raise head and shoulder. Lower. Relax.

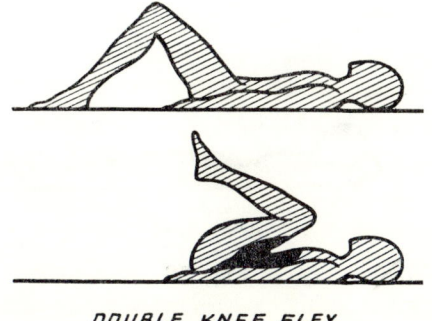

DOUBLE KNEE FLEX

Fig. 57

3. Supine "single knee kiss," knees flexed. Raise head and one knee trying to bring head as close to knee as possible. Return to starting position. Alternate knees.
4. Supine "double knee flex." Bring both flexed knees to chest. Lower. Relax. (Fig. 57).
5. Supine "double knee kiss," knees flexed. Raise head and shoulder and both knees simultaneously, trying to bring head and knees as close together as possible.
6. "Sit up." Starting position as above with knees flexed. Therapist holds feet. Sit up. Assist as necessary. Hands clasped behind neck—if patient is too weak, keep hands beside body, later cross over chest.

Strengthening for Hip Flexors
1. Supine, legs straight. Bring up knee to chest with resistance given above knee.
2. "Sit up." Sit up with straight legs. Legs held by therapist.
3. Heel slide. Patient lying on back, hands locked behind head, bend both knees, bring heels towards buttocks, slowly slide heels away from buttocks, keeping back pressed against table throughout exercise. Relax. (Fig. 58).

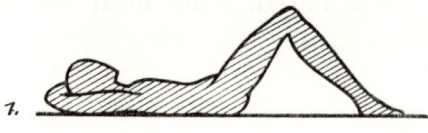

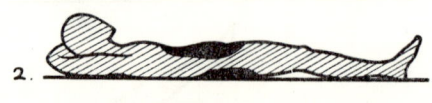

HEEL SLIDE
Fig. 58

Strengthening for Back Muscles
1. Prone. Single straight leg raising. (Fig. 59).

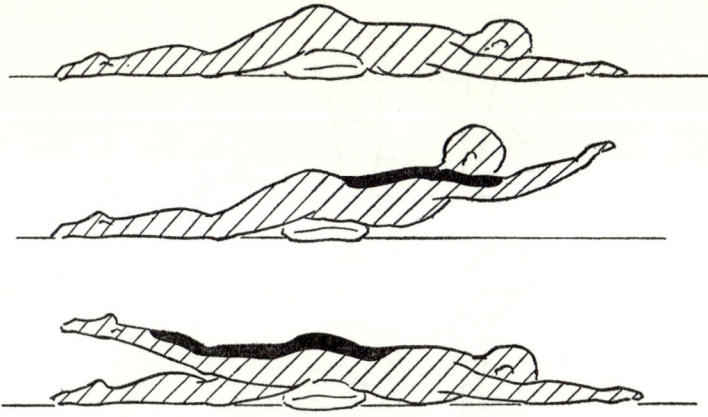

PRONE SINGLE ARM-LEG RAISE
Fig. 59

2. Prone. Single straight arm raising. (Fig. 59).
3. Prone. Raise left arm and straight right leg. Alternate. Use pillow under chest if difficult. (Fig. 59).
4. Prone. Tighten gluteal muscles. Relax.
5. Prone, pillow under hips. Raise chest holding hands behind neck. Relax.
6. Prone, pillow under hips. Raise both straight legs.

Stretching for Hamstring and Back Muscles

1. Lie supine, both knees flexed. Flex hip as much as possible then extend knee until pull of muscle is felt, lower slowly. Always maintaining enough stretch of hamstring muscles. Alternate legs. The same exercise performed with ankle in maximum dorsi flexion will stretch calf muscle.
2. Supine, inactive leg flexed, active leg straight. Raise leg slowly with knee straight as high as possible. Alternate. With ankle in dorsi flexion this exercise will stretch calf muscle.

These two exercises should be preceded by giving resistance to respective movements. In resistance exercises no feeling of stretch should be noticed.

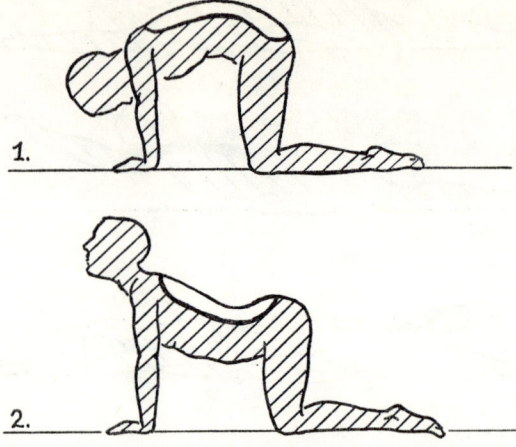

CAT'S BACK
Fig. 60

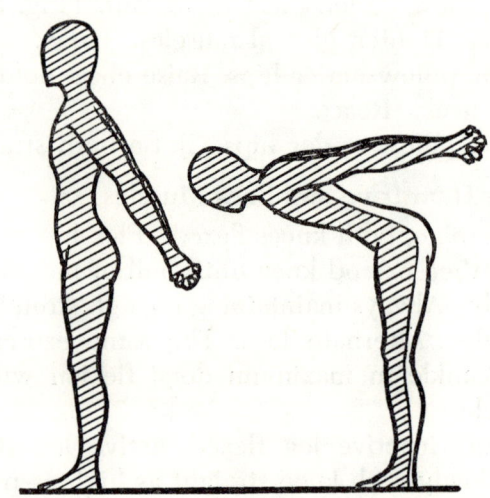

STANDING STRETCH - ARMS BACK - TO AVOID ROUND BACK

Fig. 61

Musculo-Skeletal Apparatus

3. Catback. Assume knee-hand position. Curve back like a cat, pulling in stomach, bend head—then arch back, extend head. (Fig. 60).
4. Hamstring stretch standing: Stan, clasp hands behind back, bend from hip keeping straight until you feel pull in hamstrings.
5. Calf muscle stretch standing. Stand 10" from table. Support yourself on table with hands, arms stretched out. Lean forward towards table keeping heels on the floor.
6. Floor touch: Patient is requested to stand straight, feet close together, then relax and "hang" his trunk and neck forward from the hips. After having assured relaxation, a patient should stretch down as far as he can, now stretching relaxed back and hamstring muscles.

These exercises should be started gradually. The program is written out at the beginning of the treatment and a gradual increase of exercises in order of severity is provided.

It is desirable to alternate supine and prone exercises to avoid stiffening of muscles. This may call for the use of exercises as "fill ins" even when they are not demanded by the muscle test.

1. We like to start this exercise program by having patient

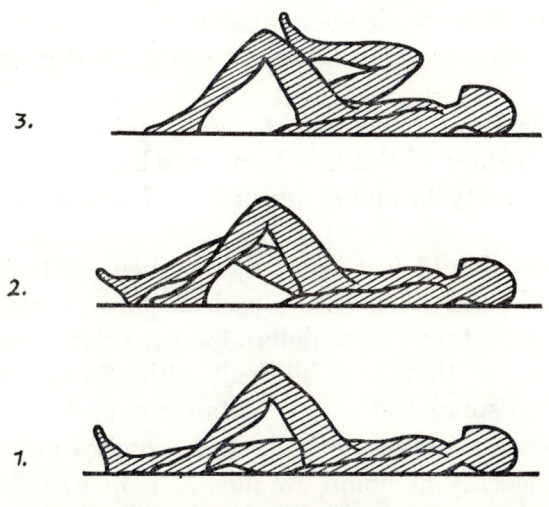

FLEXION — EXTENSION OF HIP AND KNEE — LYING

Fig. 62

lie in a supine position with pillow over knees and a roll of towels under the head and have him breath deeply and exhale slowly through pursed lips using this period of breathing to relax the patient.

2. Supine, knees flexed. Bring alternating knees to chest. Return to starting position. Extend, sole sliding. Return to starting position again. (Fig. 62).

3. Side lying, legs relaxed with knees semi-flexed. Slide upper knee towards chest. Return to starting position. Relax. Repeat two or three alternating sides.

4. Prone gluteal setting.

Acute Back Pain

Acute back pain occurs frequently after heavy-lifting, sudden movements such as twisting or fast stooping, or combined stooping and lifting, exposure to chills, fatigue or maintaining of forced position over a prolonged period of time. Sometimes the acute episode does not set in at once, but is preceded by increasing pain and tenderness for several days.

Common occurrences mentioned in histories are outdoor work in spring after lack of exercise, moving furniture, or unaccustomed heavy exertion, and, use of a soft mattress. Postural deficiencies such as weak abdominal muscles, increased lumbar lordosis, flat feet, etc., may represent other predisposing circumstances.

The typical onset consists of acute, sudden, stabbing pain in one or both sides of the low back muscles, followed by more pain, lack of ability to move, and a forced stooped and twisted position.

Treatment should first relieve pain, then gradually attempt to gain normal elasticity of back muscles. Only later should there be a complete posture test to determine pre-existent weakness or muscle tightnesses that must be dealt with. Surface anesthetics (ethyl chloride spray and use of tentanizing and sinusoidal currents) combined with gentle limbering exercises and hot packs, the latter especially at home, frequently help to relieve spasm. Bedrest may be required.

The exercises described last are used:

The patient is advised to change positions frequently, to not stand, walk or sit too long and to do the above exercises once or twice on the half hour. If radiation of pain to thigh, but no neurological symptoms are present, one should think of triggerpoint in tensor fasciae or gluteal muscles.

Frequently patients cannot be treated successfully with surface anesthetics and exercises because they live too far from the place of treatment because they are unwilling even temporarily to give up their present occupation. It is then illogical to postpone hospitalization until operation is being debated, and a fair trial with early or immediate rest at home or hospital, with surface anesthetics, may often be the means of avoiding much longer bed rest and more drastic measures.

When pain subsides a muscle test, as indicated before, will be given. If back is a "muscular" low back (that is, if no major pathology is present) further treatment will consist mainly of exercises based on the muscle test. The dosage of exercises should be increased very slowly, especially if there is considerable weakness. Stretching exercises should be postponed until trunk strength approaches normal. Pain may have to be followed with surface anesthetics. Gradually the exercises will be done three, or only two, times daily but for more extended periods. One halfhour a day is necessary.

Supportive physical therapy will include use of sinusoidal current to relieve muscle tightness and tenderness; deep kneading massage and deep effleurage for the same indications are especially useful in patients who do not too well tolerate sinusoidal current; at a later stage rolling massage for fibrositis, mecholyl or histamine iontophoresis for "jelling pain" may be necessary. Ethyl chloride spray will be useful throughout the treatment to lessen discomfort and relieve spasm. Correction of working habits and postural habits, use of firm mattresses and boards and management of emotional and situational stresses are part of a comprehensive treatment program. Triggerpoints may have to be injected as they occur.

Fractures of lumbar or thoracic vertebrae without neurological complications and without involvement of pedicles, can be mobilized frequently without the use of plaster corsets or braces. Mobilization does not mean immediate ambulation, and sitting may be tolerated even later than standing. Exercises are started in prone and supine positions from the first day, if possible. Use of hard mattress on hard board is essential.

The exercises for the first few days may be the same as used for acute back pain and should be supported by use of ethyl chloride spray. As the patient improves, the exercises should gradually increase and include gentle abdominal strengthening and back muscle strengthening exercises. They should first be given frequently during the day and for very short periods only; turning over from prone to supine position repeatedly may be the first exercise given. Limbering and strengthening exercises should be followed by stretching exercises only later when the patient has been able to get up and to walk around without difficulties. Even then stretching should be started very gently and well within pain limits. Once the patient has no pain and is ready for muscle test, exercises will be based on test results.

If immobilization in plaster jacket or in brace is necessary, exercises should start immediately, as soon as tolerated, while the patient is in plaster, and strengthening exercises can progress faster. Stretching of hamstrings to compensate for stiffness of back muscles is important and should be started from the beginning. When trunk support is discontinued, rest periods during the day will be necessary and exercises will have to be reduced to very mild limbering exercises and increased only as tolerated. Transition from back support to full activity and to full exercise program should be very gradual to avoid straining of weak and stiff muscles.

As mentioned before, prone and supine exercises should be frequently alternated. We find it helpful to start the patient with two exercises at the most and add one or two each session. The patient is instructed to remember the sequence of the exercises as well as the exercises themselves and to do them in proper sequence and then in reverse, thereby achieving a "warm-up," "work-out" and "cool-off" order. Each exercise should be performed two or three times and, as long as there are only a few exercises given, can be repeated as a whole group until the time limit is reached.

THE NECK

Acute

Acute muscle strain in the neck region may affect the neck muscles proper or the trapezius, as well as other muscles of the upper back or upper dorsal spine, causing pain and inability to move the neck.

The history will frequently include chills in neck, back and shoulder regions, sudden movements of the head, especially after holding it in a fixed position for a long time, such as at movies or when writing. Sudden passive jerking of the head such as produced by car collisions ("whiplash" injuries) is another frequent cause of acute muscle strain in the neck. More often than not these injuries occur to persons who have tense shoulder girdle and neck muscles and a vicious cycle between pain and tension makes management difficult.

If the scaleni are affected, pain may radiate to the upper extremity. Treatment is by surface anesthetics for the painful area and exercises on the half hour. Tetanizing and sinusoidal currents can be very helpful if well tolerated. Hot packs can be used at home and medication with tranquilizers and spasm-relieving drugs may be necessary. Exercises will stress relaxation and limbering as well as gentle stretching movements:

1. Pull up shoulders and let go. Relax.
2. Head rotation with and without gentle resistance and stretch.
3. Flexion/Extension of head.
4. Tilting of head, gentle resistance and stretch.

Movements should be accompanied by use of Ethyl Chloride spray to relieve pain.

Sometimes traction and collars must be prescribed, especially if the acute condition has not been detected at an early stage. Before any therapy is started, it is imperative to have good x-rays of the cervical spine. Overlooking possible bone lesion (such as fracture or dislocation of a vertebra or tuberculosis) may obviously have extremely serious results in the cervical region.

Chronic

Chronic tightness and pain of neck and shoulder girdle muscles follow acute trauma, but more often than not are due to tension. The irritant may be extrinsic and occupational or situational or intrinsic, emotional only. Frequently both are combined. Working posture and assuming of cramped position are important factors and supportive prescription will have to deal with these postural and occupational hazards as well as consider eye sight and lighting. X-rays frequently show osteoarthritic changes narrowing of disc interspaces but severity of complaints often is not related to these findings. Often marked x-ray changes are observed in completely asymptomatic necks.

As in low back prescriptions, the presence of skin tenderness calls for fibrositis massage; deep tenderness in the muscles requires deep point massage; acute painful limitation of motion should be treated with surface anesthetics and exercise.

Typical triggerpoints can be often found in sub-occipital area at the cranial insertion of the sternomastoid muscle, in trapezius muscles and upper rhomboids. Triggerpoints in supra and infraspinatus may produce radiation of pain to arm simulating nerve root compression. Exercises will again stress limbering, relaxing and gentle stretching. Passive stretching by traction should only be used if no acute spasm is present since acute spasm frequently does not respond well to this method of treatment. Traction in the lying position is usually superior to sedentary traction. In cases where actual nerve root compression exists, traction and use of collar are important parts of the treatment and if actual herniation of disc is present, they are frequently the only means for a conservative attempt.

In chronic neck pain it is necessary to develop the habit of frequent shoulder shrugging and head-turning (e.g. whenever rising from and sitting down at a desk, reaching for a telephone or book, etc., depending on the occupation). The patient often needs to form these habits in order to gain more than temporary relief.

Congenital Torticollis (Wry Neck)

The cause is usually birth injury to sterno-mastoid muscle. The muscle is foreshortened, tight. Rotation of the neck to the side of the injury is limited; tilting is limited to the side opposite the injured muscle.

Exercises should be started at the time diagnosis is made, that is, possibly in the very first weeks of life. They are therefore *gentle* passive exercises: Rotation through full and up to increasing range; tilting to the limited side. Positioning and carrying the infant in a manner causing corrective movement of the head is important.

As the child grows older, stretching may be done more vigorously—*never violently*. Resistance work may be added, at times, and still later. Ten to thirty minutes a day should be devoted to the exercises, 30 minutes in two 15-minute periods constituting the proper amount for a child over one year of age.

Massage to the contracted neck muscles is valuable as supportive prescription.

THE UPPER EXTREMITY

A number of factors enter into treatment of the upper extremity:

Type of Work: The type of work performed by the patient is of significance. The final aim of the treatment program differs according to whether the upper extremity of an artist or a skilled worker, or an upper extremity used for hard but less precise work, as in heavy labor, is being treated. The patient's profession not only influences this aim, and therefore the exercise program, but will have to be taken into account in accessory prescriptions.

Occupation may be a deciding factor in the question of whether support of the extremity or complete cessation of work is to be prescribed. All these considerations are equally important in a pre-operative program, or in a program following operation upon the upper extremity.

Crutch Walking: Crutch walking may be necessary after operation upon the lower extremity or following other disabling conditions of the legs. In rehabilitation of such cases, strengthening of the whole upper extremity, especially of the triceps and forearm muscles, will be helpful. Here the upper extremity will have to be trained as a temporary or permanent weight-bearing instrument.

Sleeping Position: A special problem in the treatment of injury to the upper extremity is presented by the patient's position in sleep. It is very difficult to rest a painful shoulder comfortably in a recumbent position, and especially so when the patient is in the habit of sleeping on the affected side. The use of several small pillows is suggested for such cases.

Prescription: Relief of pain is the first step when mobilizing a painful upper extremity. Ethyl chloride spray and relaxing exercises, preferably in supine position when the extremity is weak, are used.

In cronic cases pain is sometimes a minor factor, and the main emphasis may then be placed on stretching contractures and increasing muscle strength in weak muscle groups.

Muscle test, as always, will precede prescribing of the exercises. Testing may be difficult when substitution of muscle groups has taken place.

A strength-building program may require relatively slower increases in some cases and faster in others, and may be started on different levels, depending on the degree of weakness. Development of elasticity will have to encompass most phases of elasticity-building exercises, and frequently stress passive stretching.

Acute Injury to the Shoulder Girdle
Fracture of the Clavicle

In every method of treatment—whether internal or external fixation, or other—fingers, wrist and elbow should be given an opportunity to move immediately. Most of the shoulder proper should be treated likewise, as soon as feasible.

The outline below suggests exercises for fracture of a clavicle treated with figure-of-eight bandages in a person of middle age:

First Week: Exercises 1 and 2 to be performed every hour for the first two days, every two or three hours, plus Exercise 3 for the days following. The exercises should be performed sitting or standing; lying only if this is too strenuous.

1. Make a fist with hand. Touch shoulder. Return to starting position.
2. Hands clasped on stomach. Raise outstretched arms to 90°. Return to starting position.
3. Elbows flexed, thumbs touching chest. Abduct as far as comfort permits. Return to starting position.

Musculo-Skeletal Apparatus

Second Week: As above, three times daily up to ten or fifteen minutes, adding Exercises 4 and 5 below pain limits.
  4. Abduct arms, thumbs toward ceiling. Arms back to thighs.
  5. Same as 4, with thumbs toward floor.

Third and Fourth Weeks: Exercises 1 through 4, plus same exercises with a weight of one pound quickly increased to tolerance. Add:
  6. Crawl with fingers of right hand from umbilicus to forehead and back. Repeat on left side (Fig. 63).

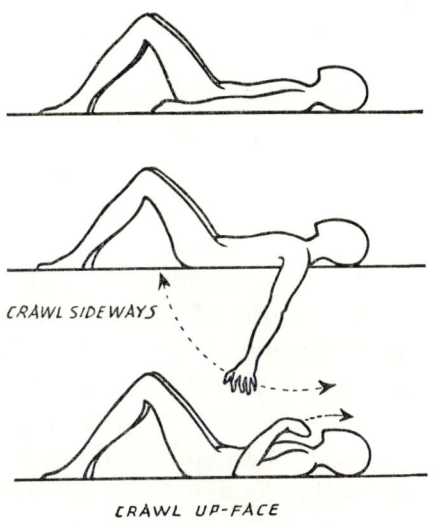

Fig. 63

  7. Touch neck with palm of right hand. With left hand. Alternate.

Exercise periods should be increased to two fifteen-minute sessions daily.

After bony union and removal of bandages, following exercises of the shoulder may be performed. Add:
  8. Touch back as high as possible with back of right hand, left hand. Alternate.
  9. Hands clasped at nape of neck (Fig. 64). Push elbows as far back as possible. Relax. Repeat.

10. Hands clasped. Raise arms as high as possible without bending forward.

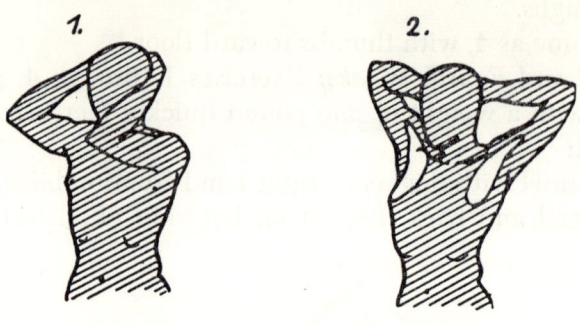

PECTORAL STRETCH
Fig. 64

The problem on removal of the bandage will be shortening of adductors and rotators of the shoulder, weakness of adductor elevators and rotators of the shoulder joint. There ought not to be any weakness or shortening of the arm or any of the other muscles of the upper extremity, because the previously outlined program should have kept them close to full function.

As soon as these exercises can be performed with some degree of success, Exercise 10 should be done, holding a rod or cane being substituted for joining hands, thereby giving more gravity to the elevation. From the start, all shoulder exercises should be done against resistance, and gentle reflex stretching of shortened muscles should be carried out. The program should be widened by increasing weight and by adding further exercises.

The home schedule at this point should extend to at least one half-hour period daily. When it is desirable to speed up the pace, the schedule may even include a half-hour twice a day. While young and active individuals will need instruction only, older people may require regular and consistent exercise sessions.

Fracture of the Head of the Humerus

Depending on the type of fracture (impacted with or without dislocation and on the type of fixation or reduction used, the period of immobility of the shoulder joint proper varies between immediate mobilization (in cases of well-impacted fractures of neck of the humerus or hairline fractures) and several weeks of immobilization (in cases requiring surgery or fixation after reduction).

In almost all cases, however, hand, wrist and fingers should be kept at full function from the start. In the majority of cases it will be possible to keep the muscles of the elbow joint near full function within the first week with the following exercise:

> Arms at sides, elbows extended. Make a fist. Touch shoulder. Return to starting position.

Shoulder exercises, if permissible from the start, should consist of very gentle passive flexion and extension, well within pain limits for the first day or two, followed by gentle abduction with the hand of therapist guarding and guiding the full length of the humerus toward the end of the first and the beginning of the second week.

The following exercises will be given gradually, with resistive-assistive exercises, as soon as the condition of the fracture warrants:

1. Supine, touch shoulder with fist, extend.
2. Supine, bring arm to chest, abduct elbow slowly.
3. Supine, hands clasped on stomach. Raise extended arms overhead to pain limit. Return to starting position.

At a more advanced stage:

4. Supine, bring up arm straight and return to side of chest.
5. Bend elbow, bring arm across chest, return to side.
6. Standing, touch neck.
7. Standing, touch back.

Resistance and assistance should always be adapted to tolerance of patient, and ethyl chloride spray frequently used to relieve pain. It should be carefully watched that the movement be scapulo-humeral rather than scapulo-thoracic.

Movement against gravity or resistance should not be given before the patient is able to perform without substitution. Premature overloading will produce loss of scapulo-humeral motion and "freezing" of shoulder joint. Poorly performed pulley exercises or pendulum exercises or wall climbing are often responsible for contractures of the shoulder joint.

Once shoulder motion is possible against gravity, weight

lifting exercises should be added and follow the previously discussed principle of gradual increase of overload.

The problems, once bony union has been established, are similar to those in mobilization of a shoulder joint after fracture of the clavicle.

Injury to the muscles of the shoulder joint or their attachment may complicate the problem. This simply means postponing rather than changing the type of exercises required for strength and elasticity of the affected muscles. In later stages, if shoulder joint cannot be mobilized in time to prevent contracture of adductors and rotators, passive stretching may have to be added. The use of deep heat and massage at this point is sometimes an aid as an accessory prescription.

Achromio-Clavicular Dislocation

This injury is sometimes treated by surgery—wiring of the joint or use of fascia for suture of the joint. Sometimes immediate mobilization is preferred.

Surgical procedure will require immobilization for some time and the main emphasis should be placed on preserving strength and mobility of the upper extremity from the upper arm downward. Exercises follow the previous pattern.

In cases of immediate mobilization a sling should be employed for support during the first week and, if necessary, the second. Exercises will stress strengthening of the shoulder muscles and avoiding of contractures.

The use of surface anesthetics will be necessary in early stages. Without operation immobilization of the shoulder joint is of no advantage.

Dislocation of the Shoulder Joint

After reduction, the immediate aim is to preserve elbow and hand strength and mobility. As soon as shoulder motion is permitted, the objective should be strengthening the inward and outward rotators and the deltoid muscle:

Exercises should stress resistance and building of muscle strength in a limited range especially if the dislocation occurred in a younger individual and was a first traumatic dislocation.

Abduction and elevation should not extend beyond 80 degrees until good strength has been obtained and the younger the patient, the longer one might wait with exercises aiming at increase of range.

Attempt to avoid recurrent dislocations by strengthening exercises is unsuccessful.

Post-operatively, exercises to strengthen shoulder muscles and restore range are needed to obtain optimum results.

Acute Bursitis of the Shoulder

Acute Bursitis of the Shoulder is characterized by acute onset of severe pain and limitation of motion in the shoulder joint, with no history of acute trauma. Frequently there is a period of more or less severe discomfort preceding the acute attack, and sometimes a history of occupational strain can be found.

Pain is usually located in the region of the head of the humerus. Abduction and elevation are painful, as well as inward and outward rotation of the shoulder. X-ray may or may not show the presence of calcium deposits near the major or minor tuberosity of the humerus.

Various procedures are used for this condition, some of them being: injection of hydrocortone and procaine, x-ray therapy, incision and removal of any calcium deposit present. The use of surface anesthetics plus immediate active motion has been found very satisfactory in many cases. This method should always be tried for two to four days, before resorting to less conservative ones.

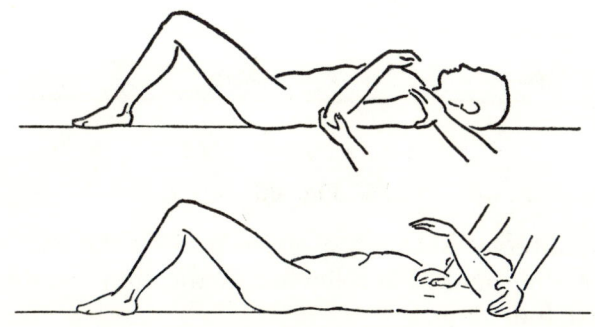

GUIDED ABDUCTION OF SHOULDER

Fig. 65

Novocaine iontophoresis of a large area of the shoulder, including the scapula, trapezius and pectoral region, as well as the upper arm to the elbow joint, may be used. If ethyl chloride spray is employed, a smaller area should be treated first, and the area increased as the pain migrates. Use guided exercises (Fig. 65).

Triggerpoints can produce acute attacks of shoulder pain. Once spasm has been relieved and triggerpoints can be palpated, they should be injected.

Exercises should first consist of gentle support and guided movement:

1. Touch shoulder.
2. Abduction with hand on chest. Usual sitting since supine position is frequently poorly tolerated. Once acute pain has subsided, exercises 3-6 should be added:
3. Supine, hands clasped on stomach. Raise outstretched arms over head to pain limit. Return to starting position (Fig 66).

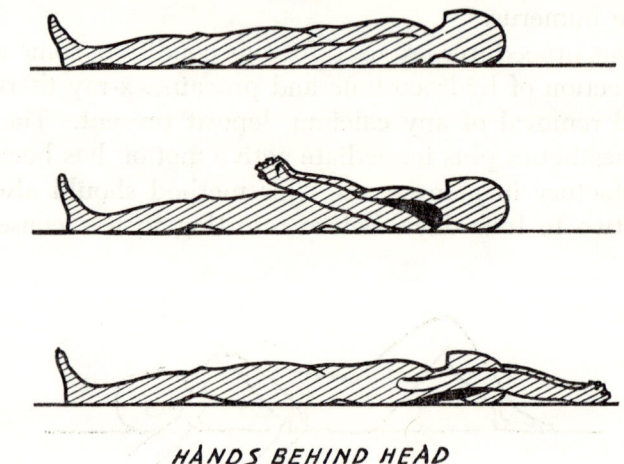

HANDS BEHIND HEAD
Fig. 66

In the interval between exercise periods the arm should be rested in a sling and pain-relieving medication should be given for the first four days.

4. Supine. Abduct arms. Slide arms back to thighs.
5. Supine. Crawl with fingers of one hand toward forehead from umbilicus and return to starting position. Alternate hands.

6. Standing. Touch neck with palm of alternate hands.

7. Standing. Touch back as high as possible with back of alternate hands.

The number of exercise periods should be reduced to once an hour and once every two hours on the third and fourth days.

After the fourth day the sling may usually be discarded temporarily and should, if possible, be permanently discarded after the first week, unless further use is desirable to prevent the patient from resuming normal activities too soon. These exercises will be added after pain has subsided:

9. Standing, hands clasped at nape of neck. Push elbows as far as possible.

10. Standing, hands clasped behind back. Lift arms as high as possible without bending forward.

11. Standing, hand on back. Crawl up with fingers toward shoulder blades, without bending forward.

Later resistance is added.

Operative removal of calcium as in the acute stage is sometimes helpful but should be followed by exercises and combined with pain-relieving supportive prescription for maximum relief in the shortest time.

As soon as no further increase of range can be obtained by this procedure and acute pain is relieved, gradually increasing passive stretching should be added.

Pendulum exercises, gibbet exercises and pulley exercises are often used, as well as the "wall-crawling" exercises, but have been found less effective, and sometimes harmful.

Chronic Bursitis of the Shoulder

Chronic bursitis of the shoulder may either be the outcome of an acute bursitis or have a history of gradually increasing discomfort, very frequently due to an occupational background, poor sitting habits and poor ways of lying. An important cause again is tension.

Triggerpoints are frequently present and so is fibrositis especially of trapezius. Adequate treatment requires consideration of all these findings. Supportive prescription must include detailed instructions as to work, posture, sleeping and sitting habits and management of tension.

Exercise given as in acute bursitis; but resistive and stretching exercises are usually in order from the start.

Acute Injury to the Muscles of the Shoulder

Acute strain of the shoulder muscles may be due to sudden jarring of the shoulder, pulling of an arm when trying to hold on to a banister to prevent a fall, throwing of a ball or javelin, etc.

Partial tears or strains of the affected muscles frequently recover with a regime of surface anesthetics and half-hour scattered exercises. (See Exercises 1 through 12 under Acute Bursitis.) In severe cases rest in a sling is sometimes added to such a regime. For very severe cases (complete tear of the muscles of the semi-tendenous cuff), operative repair may be necessary. In the acute stage, spasm and subsequent contracture will have to be dealt with. Weakness may only become a problem at a later stage.

Chronic Muscle Injury of the Shoulder may follow acute trauma. Treatment follows that outlined in Chronic Bursitis.

Fracture of the Shaft of the Humerus

Most fractures of the shaft of the humerus entail temporary immobilization of the elbow and shoulder joints or, at least, restriction of movement in these joints for some time. Surgical procedures vary from "hanging plaster," a bandage that serves mainly as a traction device, to operative fixation or complete external immobilization in a plaster jacket reaching to the wrist.

The first aim here is to maintain full finger motion and strength and full wrist motion whenever possible.

When the condition of the fracture allows full training of the extremity, the main problems will be weakness of abductors and rotators of the shoulder. Follow up the above program with resistive and assitive exercises, again starting as soon as possible and concentrating on the elbow.

Fracture of the Distal End of the Humerus and Intra-Articular Fractures of the Elbow Joint

Immediate use of the fingers is possible. Use of the wrist for supination and use of the shoulder joint may be delayed, depending on the type of fracture present. Exercises should follow the preceding outline.

Mechanical obstacles to full elbow motion, such as adhesions, interposition of fragments or incomplete results of reduction may produce complications. It will be useless to try to overcome mechanical obstacles formed by bone structures. Contractures of the joint capsule, however, can sometimes be stretched passively. The muscle should be thoroughly warmed up and always participate in the stretch, to avoid injury to muscle and tendon proper.

Elbow Joint Dislocations

Quick mobilization after reduction is highly important. The fear of myositis ossificans does not seem to be warranted if, in the earlier stages, the immediate mobilization is carried on below pain and fatigue limits. If immobilized, full range and strength of shoulder joint, of wrist (if possible) and certainly of all fingers, should be preserved.

After immobilization, graded exercises should be directed primarily toward lengthening the elbow muscles and secondarily toward strength. If mobilization is tried, early surface anesthetics may be needed to make mobilization more effective. The exercise program again starts with scattered dosage and gradually increases to more prolonged but fewer periods of exercise. In later stages, as always in the treatment of the upper extremity, the patient's profession will have an important bearing on deciding whether increases of strength or increase of range ought to be stressed.

Acute sprains of the elbow joint are not very common. Both acute and chronic injuries of the elbow joint are related chiefly to the muscular-tendonous apparatus, if there are no fractures or major tears of the ligament.

Chronic Injury to the Elbow Region
Tennis Elbow

This common condition is encountered not only, as the name suggests, among tennis players, but as the result of faulty use of the affected extremity in any recurrent stereotyped movement. Turning door knobs, carrying weights, handling telephones, closing elevator doors, etc., may all produce pain in the lower arm and elbow region with main focus in the elbow. Permanent relief is unlikely unless the cause—the faulty movement—is found, and either corrected or eliminated. In tennis a top-spin in the serve, a backhand executed with a twist of the wrist, too small a racket handle, or various other details, may produce the pain.

There are different "types" of tennis elbow: the common symptom is usually pain upon dorsiflexion of the wrist with clenched fist and extended forearm. The pain occurs usually in the forearm. There may or may not be pain and tenderness at the condyle proper and painful tenderness of the muscle bellies of the forearm. Pain alone may be present with no tenderness at all upon motion and possibly some limitation of motion.

Cases with tenderness and pain at the humerus condyle may require injection of hydrocortone into periosteum. Cases with tenderness in the muscle belly require deep massage. Injection of triggerpoint followed by local spasm-relieving physical therapy may be needed. If tenderness of forearm muscles without triggerpoint is present, kneading massage, sinusoidal current, ethyl chloride spray are helpful.

Fracture of the Forearm

Retaining function in the shoulder joint and fingers is possible in most methods of fixation and most types of fracture. The elbow (Ex. 9, 10) may be free only at later stages. This mobility should be utilized fully by immediate exercises.

1. Close fist. Open and fan out fingers. Keep thumb inside fist.
2. Same as 1, with thumb outside of fist.
3. Grasp small sponge or rubber ball and squeeze. (Limitation of this exercise has been described, *see* page 168.)
4. Bend and stretch fingers against resistance.
5. Bend and stretch fingers against increased resistance.
6. Touch thumb with index finger. Stretch index finger. Repeat with other fingers.
7. Touch neck with fist.
8. Touch back with fist.
9. Flex and extend elbow.
10. Hand on opposite shoulder. Supinate. Pronate (Fig. 67.)

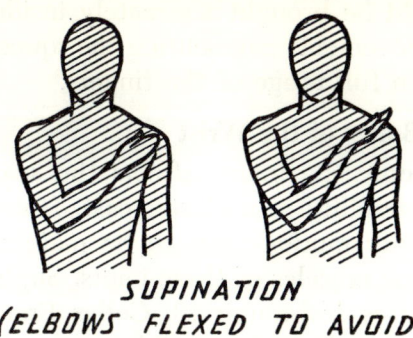

SUPINATION
(ELBOWS FLEXED TO AVOID
SHOULDER MOTION)
Fig. 67

The main problems after complete removal of fixation will be: weakness of elbow flexion, extension and supination; weakness of wrist flexion, extension and supination; contracture of elbow flexors, extensors and supinators; and contracture of wrist flexors, extensors and sometimes supinators. Exercises for the wrist should be stressed. Increasing resistance to the shoulder and elbow, as well as stretching of the latter, should be given.

Fracture of Distal End of Radius
Colles Fracture

In less severe cases, shoulder, elbow and fingers will be free for immediate treatment with exercises 1-10 described above. Weights and resistance should be employed beginning with the second week.

In more severe cases the elbow is often immobilized for some time. Never neglect the maintenance of full finger motion and strength and of full shoulder motion and strength.

It is a great mistake to allow function to deteriorate in fingers and shoulder. This is especially true in older people when mobility of these joints (restoration of normal muscle elasticity) creates a serious and totally unnecessary problem, often long after the actual injury has healed. Another frequent error is made in the prescription of the "rubber ball" exercise. If the patient is advised to squeeze a rubber ball, he will exercise the joints of his finger in a limited way only. He should be told to close the fist tightly and then open it until the fingers are maximally stretched.

The thumb should be brought alternately inside and outside of the fist. These movements augmenting the squeezing of a rubber ball help maintain full range of the fingers.

Injury to Small Bones of the Wrist

Most commonly the injury affects the scaphoid bone and requires long immobility in a plaster cast. However, full finger, elbow and shoulder motion have to be maintained, as well as full strength of the muscles of these joints. Supination and pronation (see Exercises 1 through 10, Colles Fracture) should be started immediately whenever possible.

After removal of the plaster, there must be in addition strengthening of wrist (flexion, extension and supination) as well as regaining full thumb motion (in scaphoid lesions, the first phalanx of the thumb must be immobilized).

Acute trauma to the wrist, resulting in "sprain," is much less frequent than fracture to the small bones, mainly the scaphoid. X-rays are imperative, and the diagnosis "sprained wrist" should be made, if at all, with extreme caution. In doubtful cases, and if surface anesthetics do not very markedly relieve pain, immobilization of the wrist is the method of choice. The first aim is to preserve finger, elbow and shoulder motion and strength, by means of the previously described exercises.

Chronic Conditions of the Wrist Joint

In chronic arthritis of various origin, painful limitation of wrist motion is frequent, and requires immediate or temporary immobilization. In this period exercises should try mainly for full range of the other non-affected joints of the extremity with a scattered exercise program as described on page 48.

Power building should be attempted only within the full range of the joints.

When motion is permitted again, range will be of more importance than strength, unless it is decided, on the basis of x-ray and clinical findings, that it will be doubtful whether range can be maintained beyond a certain degree. If this last is so, it is better to try to preserve supination and pronation of the joint rather than flexion and extension. A limited degree of flexion-extension or permanent fixation in slight dorsiflexion will produce a good functional hand, if combined with some supination. Once a limitation of motion has been accepted, more attention should be paid to preserving and increasing strength.

Fracture of Metacarpal Bones

Occasionally complete motion of the whole extremity can be maintained from the beginning of treatment. In some cases the fingers of the affected bone may be temporarily immobilized. Maintaining full range of the unaffected joints is again the first consideration: see Exercises 7 through 10 in the preceding section on the **Wrist.**

When fixation has been removed, mobilization of immobilized fingers and strength-building exercises are to be emphasized.

Resistive-assistance exercises are important. To scatter dosage is equally so, since small muscles with relative weakness do not lend themselves to massive strength-building dosage as quickly as the larger, more powerful muscles of the rest of the upper extremity.

Fracture of the Fingers

Immobilization of fingers should be avoided whenever possible, because mobilization of the small joints is especially difficult after prolonged rest.

Sprains are frequent and should be treated with immediate mobilization, preferably with the aid of ethyl chloride spray. Immobilization of sprained fingers usually leads to longer disability, and in older people may create permanent disability of the fingers involved. The pertinent exercises are, as previously described, opening and closing fists with thumb inside and out; and bending and stretching fingers against resistance; also wringing out a wet towel and flexing the individual fingers.

Flexion or extension of each individual fingerjoint as well as abduction and adduction should be exercised with resistance, stretch, and assistance as needed. Home exercises should be carried out for short periods every ½ hour and for longer periods 2-3 times a day. A cooperative patient can act quite efficiently as his own therapist with his uninvolved hand.

Diagnosis should consider the possible tearing of tendons, especially of extensor tendons of the fingers, a relatively frequent occurrence. A typical symptom is inability to extend the last phalanx. Immobilization or surgery will be indicated.

THE LOWER EXTREMITIES

The supportive prescription must consider especially shoes, supports or supportive bandages. *Permission to bear weight on the injured extremity is dependent not only on the ability of the structure* (bone, ligament) *to stand strain and weight bearing, but it is equally important to consider strength and flexibility of of muscles.*

IT IS A COMMON MISTAKE TO GIVE A PATIENT EARLY PERMISSION TO WALK WITH FULL WEIGHT BEARING AS MUCH AS HE WANTS AS SOON AS INJURY IS HEALED AND READY TO SUPPORT THE BODY WEIGHT. The suggestion "Walk one block today, and one block more each day until it is possible to walk as much as you want" is equally inadequate. Specific instruction is always needed when treating patient after injury. It is especially important after injury to the lower extremities. Once full weight-bearing is permitted, unconscious grading cannot be practised by the patient, as in the upper extremities.

Walking means walking on both legs. Once a patient feels discomfort, strain or fatigue in either leg, he is past the fatigue limit, and if he does not stop walking immediately, he will use the extremity poorly. A limping, awkard gait usually leads to spasm, contracture and persistent bad walking habit. Contracture in itself can be so severe as to produce permanent disability.

Another consideration in evaluating and rehabilitating the lower extremities is that of the patient's relative weight. A leg that would be perfectly satisfactory under normal circumstances, may be hopelessly inadequate when weakened after injury and subject to the weight gained by the patient during inactivity.

There is a stage after injury or surgery to the bone in the lower extremities, when the bone or joint is perfectly ready for full weight-bearing; *but* this moment rarely coincides with that at which the muscles are adequately equipped for the job.

Exercises should prepare the muscles for this time. The optimum would be to have the patient muscularly ready for full weight bearing the moment the structure is strong enough for the task. This will rarely be possible and if the muscle is too weak and not endurant enough to have the patient return to full normal activities, use of crutches, use of partial weight bearing will have to be continued. Weight bearing should never be carried past pain limits.

It is obvious that the return of patient to "normal activities" depends very much on what these activities are. In sedentary occupation return to full work will be possible much sooner than in a patient who has to do manual labor or who engages in sports, dancing, etc. In a sedentary person exercises will not necessarily have to aim at full return of function. In persons who expose themselves to re-injury by their work and other physical activities, return to full strength and flexibility is needed and exercises, therefore, carried on much longer.

The Hip Joint
Fracture of the Neck of the Femur

Fracture of the neck of the femur is usually treated by open reduction and internal fixation. Where operation is not performed immediately, the time between injury and surgery should be used to keep the patient—usually elderly people—in good shape by strengthening the upper extremity especially triceps, for the long period of crutch walking, and by maintaining full motion of ankle joint by active motion and as much quadriceps tone as possible, by quadriceps setting and by extension of knee where possible. This can be done whether the patient is just placed between sandbags or whether he is in Russell traction. Breathing exercises and arm exercises will help to keep the patient in reasonably good condition and get him acquainted with the fact that he will have to do the work for rehabilitation, that he cannot expect to get well without effort. After surgery, exercises should start at once and include quadriceps setting, prone lying—preferably many hours a day to avoid decubitus—gluteal setting. The previously mentioned movements should be continued and active flexion/extension of knee and hip joint, first sliding, then lifting, should be done as soon as possible. Abduction—sliding, later against resistance and still later lying on side with knee straight and knee flexed — should be added; prone leg raise with knee straight and with knee flexed and finally all these exercises against resistance should be given. Gentle stretching of hip flexors in the prone position may be necessary if prone lying, gluteal setting and prone leg raising have not been started early enough to avoid flexion contracture.

Hip flexion contracture and decubiti, two important problems in the treatment of hip injury, are avoidable if prone lying, gluteal setting and prone raising are practiced soon enough.

Sitting out of bed will be frequently possible in the first two or three days and walking in parallel bars, without weight bearing, then crutch walking, should follow readily.

Depending on the stability of the fracture, rotating exercises will have to wait. Once they are permitted, rotation supine with and without resistance, rotation of leg over edge of plint with and without resistance, and rotation prone with knee flexed will follow. It should only be given as the fracture is stable enough. Another exercise helping rotation is flexion and extension of knee and hip with the leg crossed over the opposite extremity. Quadriceps strengthening should include:
1. Quadriceps setting.
2. Extension of leg over a pillow.
3. Extension of leg over edge of bed against gravity, later resistance, still later weight.

After HIP ATHROPLASTY, the same approach is used. Here an additional problem is usually weakness of abductors of hip joint. If abduction should not be desirable in the beginning, static exercises and tensing of abductors against resistance, not permitting movement, may help prevent weakness of abductors. As soon as possible: (1) abduction against resistance, (2) abduction lying on side against gravity, (3) abduction against gravity and resistance, should be practiced.

As always, repetition of these movements should be limited to four or five times with always rest permitting the muscles to relax between movements. *Excessive repetitions without rest will produce shortening and tightening of muscles and substitution.* Repeat cycle.

Musculo-Skeletal Apparatus

When the hip is surgically ready, full weight bearing should be only permitted if the patient has muscles capable of permitting normal gait. If patient is permitted to limp along without crutches, he will soon acquire limping habit and it will be very much harder to break this habit than to prevent it. Limping at this stage is more often than not due to weak abductors of hip.

Osteoarthritis of Hipjoint

Frequently requires surgery; however, conservative treatment is indicated in initial and moderately severe cases. In the very old when surgery is inadvisable, as well as in the young not ready to accept operative procedure, relief from pain and improvement of function are often possible by conservative management.

The joint is relieved from strain and the muscle from fatigue, painful spasm and contracture by rest. Hot packs, surface anesthetics and other spasm-relieving therapy are necessary for the first weeks of treatment. Triggerpoints are frequently found and should be injected before starting exercises. The exercise program will follow the previously outlined principles. It includes:

1. Supine, legs straight: Touch chest with knee. Return to starting position, heel sliding.
2. Side lying: Bring upper knee to chest. Slide down and extend. Return to starting position. Relax.
3. Supine, legs straight: Cross affected leg over good leg. Slide up toward hip. Slide down, returning to starting position (Fig. 68).

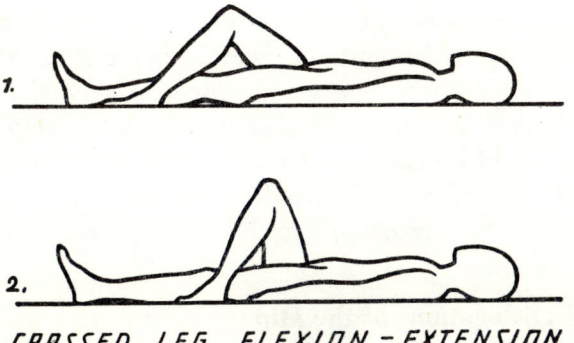

CROSSED LEG FLEXION - EXTENSION

Fig. 68

4. Do exercise 1 in this group without sliding heel.
5. Supine: Abduct leg, sliding return to starting position.
6. Prone: Tighten gluteal muscles. Relax.
7. Prone: Straight leg raising.
8. Prone: Bring heel to bottock. Lift thigh.
9. Supine, knee hanging over edge of table: Turn leg in. Turn out (Fig. 69).

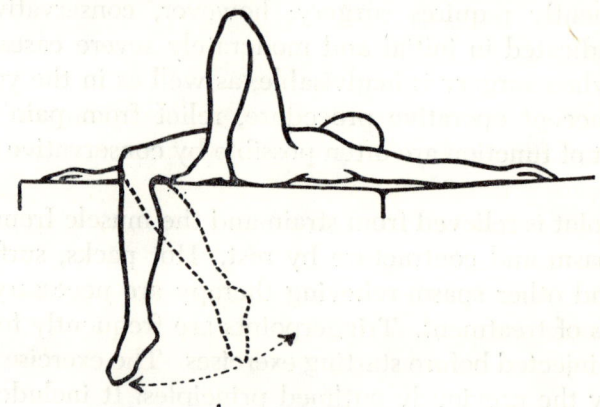

HIP ROTATION-LYING

Fig. 69

These exercises later to be given with resistance. The prone ones may require assistance for gentle passive psoas stretching. Proceed very slowly, using a surface anesthetic for pain and omitting exercises that hurt. Make sure that rest is observed and no weight bearing permitted until the release from pain is as complete as possible.

Later, deep heat (mild short wave) and massage may be used as supportive treatment, and weight-bearing exercises slowly introduced. Very short periods during the day should be increased to longer and more consistent periods of weight-bearing. Treatment should be combined with a reasonable regime of rest and exercise, as well as with avoidance of too much weight-bearing, moderatedy severe cases may be carried along for an indefinite length of time.

Congenital Dislocations of the Hip

After operation or immobilization the main problem is

strengthening of the hip rotators and sometimes contracture of inward rotators and abductors as well as the psoasiliacus. All the exercises described in this section should be given. Slow, scattered mobilization, with rest after immobilization has ended, produces better results than a forced schedule of quick weight-bearing. It is necessary in these cases to break an old habit of a waddling gait made unnecessary by successful operation and rehabilitated muscles, and to substitute correct habit forming (teaching the correct steps to be taken whenever the patient rises from a sitting position, etc.).

Acute Injuries to the Muscles of the Hip and Thigh

Acute muscle strain in the gluteal region has been described in the section dealing with low back pain, which also covered strain of the hamstrings forming part of low back, or so-called sacroiliac strain. The hip rotators and the tensor faciae latae can be strained by certain movements, especially in athletic activities. The ensuing painful limitation of motion is treated with surface anesthetics and exercises to restore muscle elasticity—all on a scattered basis.

Acute "tear" of the hamstrings frequently happens in sprinting or trying for a quick start in running. The hamstrings are pulled by quick extensor action and often respond with very acute pain and spasm. There may be a pain-free interval, but immediate limitation of motion and disability often occur. The treatment is rest, if normal walking is impossible, and immediate mobilization with the help of surface anesthetics. Strengthening exercises are usually superfluous but the following attempt to restore normal length:

1. Supine, with straight legs. Touch chest with knee. Return to starting position.
2. Same as 1. Resistance to extension for reflex stretch (Fig. 19).
3. Supine. Straight leg raising for stretch of hamstrings.
4. Prone. Knee flexion and extension. Foot should reach over edge of table to make full extension of knee possible.
5. Supine. Bring knee to chest, extend knee keeping hip flexed. Lower leg gradually as necessary to obtain full extension (Fig. 70).

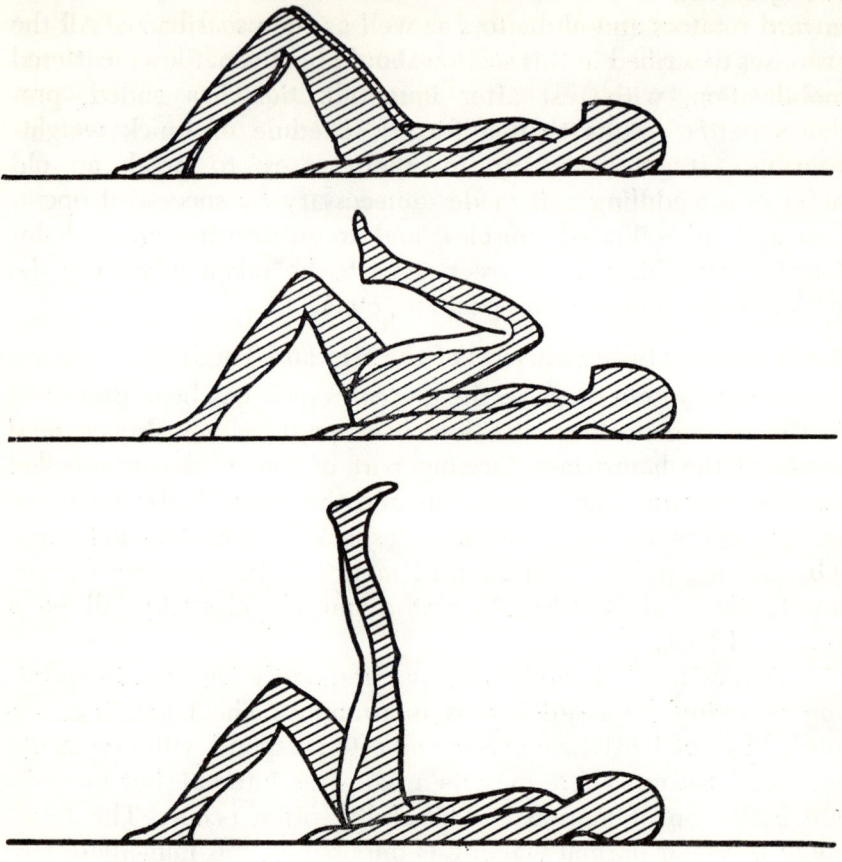

FLEXION EXTENSION FOR STRETCH

Fig. 70

6. Standing hamstring stretch. Page 116.
7. Sitting hamstring stretch. Page 116 (*Toe touch*). This exercise should be combined with use of ethyl chloride spray to raise pain threshold and be preceded by tetanizing and sinusoidal currents to painful area.

    A good athlete needs a warm-up of from one-half to a full hour to bring his muscles to maximum elasticity (this warm-up is longer than the 15 minutes found adequate experimentally (*see* Fig. 6) because it is done with slow movements). It has been seen that if a runner is flexible enough to touch the floor with his fingertips without bending his knees (*see Kraus-Weber Test,* p. 126), he is much less likely to be subject to pulling hamstrings, and this exercise should be used to prevent recurrence. Hamstring pulls due to other causes are treated similarly, always keeping in mind the patient's use of the extremity.

Chronic Strains of Hip and Thigh Muscles

Chronic strains often follow low back pain, injuries of lower extremity or foot deficiencies causing improper use of the extremity. The hip rotators may be contractured and will then require rest and active and passive lengthening. The same holds true for the tensor faciae latae.

In all cases of chronic muscle strain in the lower extremities one has to explore for triggerpoints and, if necessary, inject. Fibrositis, often present, requires rolling massage.

Fracture of the Shaft of the Femur

These fractures occur in all age groups, and do not usually involve the problem of age involved in many fractures of the neck of the femur. Hip and knee joint should be mobilized as soon as possible. Ankle and foot should be given exercises from the start to preserve strength and elasticity.

In the knee joint, when freed for motion, stress should be placed on gaining full extension, flexion to at least 90° (more if possible) and quadriceps strength. Gentle resistance, within pain and fatigue limits, and anti-gravity work should be started as soon as possible. Quadriceps setting will then be much sooner feasible. When freed for movement, the muscles of the hip joint should immediately be treated by strength-building exercises in all directions; contractures, if any, will have to be stretched, at first (if necessary) with reflex relaxation. Exercises in prone position are particularly valuable to prevent flexion-contracture of the hip joint.

If the knee shows flexion-contracture and cannot be fully extended to 180°, this should be relieved before beginning ambulation. Again, it may be advisable to use reflex stretching, passive stretching and, if necessary, weighing down the knee with sandbags, for periods during the day. Ambulation, when started, should be limited to small, scattered periods daily, and increase gradually, as previously described.

Old fractures and chronic osteomyelitis of the shaft of the femur cause chronic disabilities.

The problems involved are weakness, atrophy of the whole lower extremity from prolonged lack of use or immobilization and contracture caused by prolonged immobilization or by faulty positioning. Hip muscles frequently show flexion contracture and slight inward rotation of the femur: they require passive and active lengthening. Contractures of the hamstrings and the oblique popliteal muscle are often combined with contractures of the vastus intermedius and may produce limitation of flexion *and* extension of the knee joint at the same time.

If possible, exercises should start on a scattered basis, with the aim of establishing full hip and knee extension. (See exercises for hip and knee joints.)

Quadriceps strengthening may be done very soon and it is important to try for the last ten degrees of extension and not to permit straight leg raising before the maximum of extension has been reached. (see *Knee Joint*).

Fibrous adhesions often produce complications and may require increased passive stretching when surgically warranted. At the same time, leg and foot should receive care and here again, the aim in operative cases should be to establish a well-functioning muscle motor in time to make weight-bearing possible as soon as the surgeon allows.

It may frequently be necessary to correct old walking habits that sometimes interfere with full use of existing functional material.

In osteomyelitis, the patient's temperature needs watching. Any rise in temperature means that exercises must be stopped for muscles in proximity to the source of infection. It may be possible to continue working with leg and foot muscles when, for instance, working with thigh muscles is contra-indicated. Such possibilities should not be overlooked or neglected.

It must be remembered that walking in a plaster or walking caliper before complete mobilization has only limited exercise value for all muscles of the extremity. A period of rest without weight-bearing, and a resumption of scattered and gradually increasing exercises, should anticipate the actual start of weight-bearing. In this period too, leg and foot muscles should reach complete strength.

Fractures of the distal end of the femur are often complicated by structural blockings of the joint proper. If these are not treated by open reduction and fixation, immobilization of the knee joint at an angle below 170° will frequently be unavoidable.

The main problem after freeing the knee joint for mobilization will be flexion-contracture of the knee. Scattered exercises, first without, then against gravity, should aim at (1) lengthening knee flexors and (2) strengthening the quadriceps group.

In these fractures, contracture of the vastus intermedius often prevents satisfactory flexion of the knee joint and requires reflex-active-and-passive stretching. If exercises during fixation have kept the rest of the extremity close to normal, full attention may next be directed toward the crucial problem of strengthening the extensors of the knee joint and lengthening the foreshortened muscles. Unassisted antigravity exercises for the knee joint should not be started before the joint can be stretched to 180°, since such exercises tend to increase or to make more permanent a flexion-contracture.

A routine that suits many similar cases is the following: (1) Flexion-extension of the knee joint, either in balance suspension, with pulleys (one supporting the thigh, the other the ankle) or on a sliding board. (2) Prone flexion-extension. It is important, however, that the foot does not prevent full extension of the knee, otherwise the knee joint will not be exercised in the desired range. When the knee can be extended to the point where the foot prevents further movement, the movement should be done with the foot protruding beyond the bed or mattress. (3) Resistive-assistive exercises are especially important for this type of injury.

Knee
Fracture of the Patella

If there is no rupture of the ligamentus apparatus or dislocation of fragments, immediate mobilization may sometimes be started. The problem will be focussed mainly, in the early stages and likewise in operative cases, on maintaining the 180° extension and gaining flexion up to 90° as quickly as possible.

The first steps in treatment should try to preserve strength of the quadriceps muscle. Here as before, leg and foot muscles must not be allowed to deteriorate. Begin quadriceps setting as soon as possible. However, in some cases it is advisable to start with supported flexion-extension from 180° to 140° on a scattered basis and within pain limits. Then, as soon as surgically possible, strengthening of the quadriceps should be emphasized, and flexion pushed to 90°. Anti-gravity exercises are not to be allowed before they can be performed without loss of extension.

Intra-Articular Injuries of the Knee Joint

Injuries to the cartilage may require operation if parts of the cartilage are dislocated and block joint movements.

The use of splints or plasters does not offer any advantages, nor does the tapping of intra-articular fluid unless there is a large quantity in the joint.

If arthrotomy of the knee joint is indicated, pre-operative preparation should emphasize strengthening of the vastus medialis and, as far as the mobility of the joint is concerned, obtaining full 180° extension. Flexion to 90° should be tried for, but full extension is always more important.

Post-operatively, quadriceps setting should be started immediately. Frequently this is not possible, even if the patient has been trained before. However, in such cases flexion-extension of the knee joint in the last ten degrees, stressing extension, is sometimes possible and should then be started promptly. Straight leg raising, extension of the knee over the edge of the bed and bending and stretching against gravity should not be attempted unless the full 180° can be reached against gravity. Resistive exercises may be given from the start, but the main considerations are 180° extension and strength of the vastus medialis and quadriceps. From here on treatment follows the lines laid down for conservative handling of injuries to the knee joint.

If it is decided not to operate but to attempt conservative treatment of the injured knee joint, the procedure will be similar to that of:

Sprain, Partial Tear of Ligamentous Apparatus of the Knee Joint

As long as normal walking is not possible, patient will have to use crutches, and if there is intraarticular swelling of more than an estimated 50 cc., patient should stay off his feet. Ethyl chloride spray is used once or twice a day. Use of sinusoidal current to vastus med. and popliteus muscle is helpful. In major tears of the ligamentous apparatus and if instability can be demonstrated in x-rays, surgery may be necessary. Exercises are given for two minutes on a half-hour basis and should attempt first to reduce intra- and periarticular swellings, restore full extension and vastus medialis power. Exercises gradually increased.

1. Supine, with straight legs. Tighten quadriceps. Healthy leg is used for comparison. Relax. If patient cannot do do this, substitute: Supine, affected leg straight and held by therapist to give resistance. Bend healthy leg,

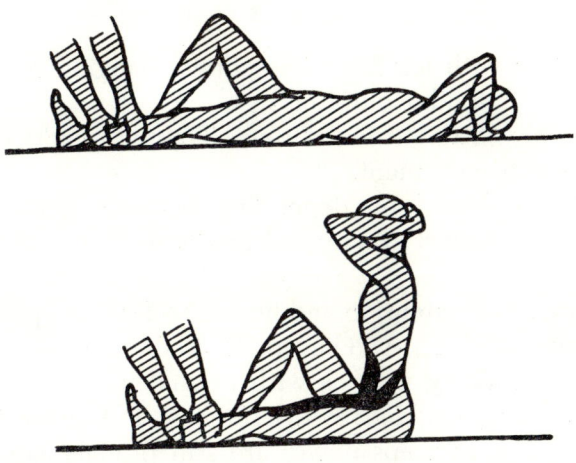

UNILATERAL SIT-UP
Fig. 71

bringing heel to buttocks. Hands behind neck, come to a sitting position. This causes reflex contraction of the quadriceps.

2. Supine. Bend knee, foot sliding, then stretch to 180° (Fig. 62).
3. Prone. Flex and extend knee. Foot is over edge of table so that toes do not interfere with full stretch.

4. Supine, with pillow under knee. Extend leg to 180°. Relax. (Fig. 72).

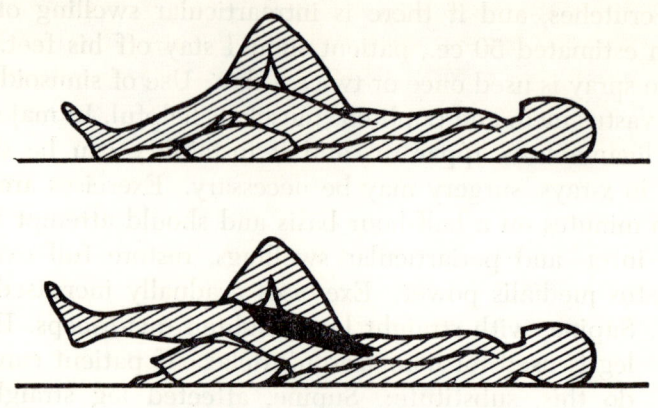

EXTENSION OVER PILLOW

Fig. 72

5. Sitting with leg from knee down hanging over edge of table. Extend. Hold. Relax.
6. Supine. Straight leg raising. Tighten quadriceps before starting movement.

(Exercises should be done, first without resistance, then with resistance, against gravity and finally weight work should be added.

As soon as full extension and flexion to 180° are possible, and intra-articular swelling is relieved, limited walking may be allowed. Short walking periods with normal use of the knee are preferable to longer periods with crutches. Full extension of the knee joint and quadriceps power are still primary aims. A secondary objective is preserving the strength and length of the other muscles of the extremity. As swelling is relieved, full extension obtained and quadriceps power improved, these exercises may be added:

7. Supine. Rotated (outward) lifting of leg in extension.

Length of exercise periods may be increased, and work against gravity started as follows:

8. Standing with feet together and hands on knees. Straighten knees, by pushing back with hands.
9. Standing with feet a foot apart. Do knee bends with

knees parallel. Get down to comfortable level, raising on toes—*do not* keep feet flat on ground and do not lower yourself completely. Relax between movements. (Contrary to some recent reports no harmful effect of this movement could be found in over 200 knee injuries followed over 20 years.)

10. Kneel. Try to sit back on heels.

Resistive-assistive exercises should be given from the start, and resistance gradually increased as assistance is diminished. As the injury improves, allow the patient to return little by little to normal work and activities. Prolonged holding of the knee in one position of the joint, such as riding in an automobile, sitting at a desk or in certain standing occupations, is unfavorable.

At night during the first few weeks a pillow under the knee may be helpful, and bandaging with an ace bandage sometimes prevents irritation from the patient's turning and twisting his leg in sleep. After good power and stability and 180°-90° range have been reached, treatment should work for the flexion not yet attained. At this point, passive stretching is sometimes necessary or advisable to lengthen the vastus intermedius.

The complete strengthening of the knee joint, particularly of the vastus medialis, is even more important than in most other joints. A knee joint that is not well protected by a strong vastus medialis is a poor risk as to recurrent injury.

As soon as gravity can be tolerated, weight can be added to the above exercises and they should be performed keeping below fatigue limits at first. Later, heavy resistance and heavy weights are indicated. It is usually possible to increase the weight twice a week, and it should be increased until full capacity for weight-lifting and satisfactory holding have been obtained.

De Lorme's method may be followed. Another way to increase weight-lifting in these cases is to add a pound or two to the weight of a sandbag, or a weight lifting boot attached to the patient's foot and to augment this weight every three days by one or two pounds. Still another method is to determine the maximum weight-lifting capacity by having the patient lift increasingly heavy weights in succession and to use the weight that can be lifted without too much effort and held without too much effort as the starting point for the above exercises. They should be given in increasingly long exercise periods, once or twice a day, preceded by warm-ups and followed by cool-offs.

A knee is not fully restored if it is not as strong as the contralateral side. While a slightly weakened knee may be satisfactory for a person whose life is mostly sedentary, restoring of full quadriceps function is a must to prevent recurrent injuries and difficulties in the knee of an athletic or of a person performing heavy physical work.

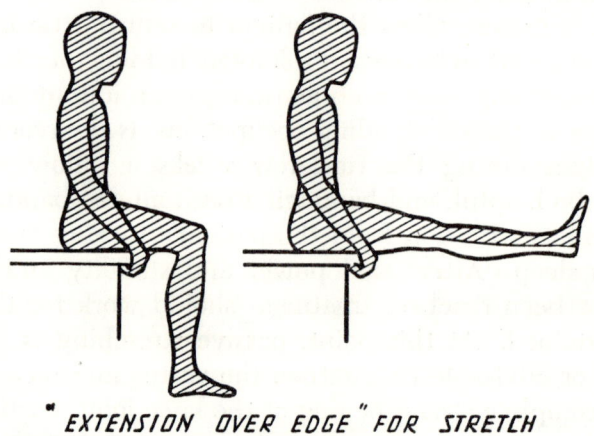

"EXTENSION OVER EDGE" FOR STRETCH OF HAMSTRINGS

Fig. 73

Chronic Conditions of the Knee Joint

Osteoarthritis: Symptoms in these knee joints often follow a history of increased weight, prolonged standing on a hard floor or forced immobilization of the knee joint through occupation. The wearing of poorly fitting shoes makes this condition especially common among elderly women.

Some limitation of flexion and extension of the knee joint is present, together with pain and tenderness on the medial side of the knee. X-rays may show "spurs" and "lipping," at times some narrowing of the joint. Knock knees, flat feet, pronated heels, fibrositis of the medial aspect of the knee joint may be present.

Treatment may require bed rest along with exercises and the daily use of surface anesthetics upon the painful area:

1. Supine. Flex, extend knee, foot sliding. Stress extension.

2. Supine. Legs straight, tighten vastus medialis.
3. Prone. Flex, extend knee. Foot is over edge of table so that it does not interfere with full stretch.
4. Prone. Place pillow under knee. Therapist assists stretching to full extension.

The main problems are contractures of oblique popliteal muscles, gastrocnemius and hamstrings. The quadriceps and especially the vastus medialis are found to be weak and to show diminished holding power. The vastus intermedius is often foreshortened. Fibrous adhesion may produce further complications. A regime of scattered exercises, adding the following to those already prescribed, emphasizes extension for vastus medialis strengthening:

5. Supine, with pillow under knee. Extend leg. Relax.
6. Supine, with leg from knee down over edge of table. Extend. Relax.
7. Supine. Straight leg raising. Tighten quadriceps before starting movement. Return. Relax. (Fig. 74).

As soon as the patient is ready for walking, that is, when he

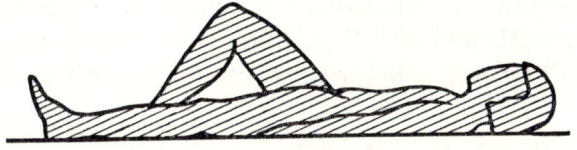

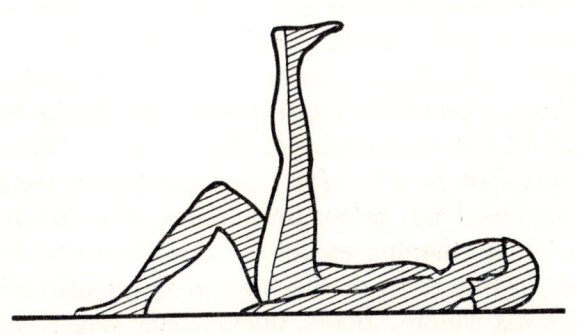

SINGLE STRAIGHT LEG RAISE FOR STRETCH OF HAMSTRINGS AND LEG MUSCLE

Fig. 74

can walk without a limp and without pain, frequent but short trips of walking may be allowed and increased little by little to longer and less frequent ones.

Return to work depends on occupation, with the possibility of part-time work to be kept in mind.

The treatment is incomplete unless repeated flexion-extension of the knee has been trained into a habit after sitting, standing or any change of position. Proper footwear, lifting of the medial side of the heel, if necessary, and supportive bandages for the leg (reaching from the foot to the tuberosity of the tibia) may be prescribed. Bandaging the knee proper is usually not beneficial. Injection of hydrocortone often relieves the symptoms but weak quadriceps remains and requires strengthening. Supportive prescriptions may include mild deep heat and histamine iontophoresis.

Fracture of the Condyles of the Tibia

This can be treated more often than not by immediate mobilization with or without balanced suspension. Since cartillage of the joint has usually suffered, weight bearing should be permitted only after several months. Muscles, especially quadriceps, should be fully strengthened and there should be a good range of knee joint and full extension before even partial weight bearing is permitted.

Fracture of the Shaft of the Tibia and Fibula

The immediate problem is maintaining strength and mobility of the non-immobilized joints. Toe exercises and strength-building exercises for the femur should be started at once, if surgically warranted. As soon as knee and ankle motion is allowed, range of knee motion from 180° to 90° should be tried for, and there should be strengthening of the anterior tibial muscles, calf muscles and foot muscles (resistive-assistive exercises).

The peroneal and soleus muscles are often contractured and need special lengthening exercises. Passive stretching may have to be added. Fractures of the leg are frequently allowed up in plaster-of-Paris walking boots, during later stages. Such walking boots reach in some cases to well above the knee joint, and in other cases extend to the tuberosity of the tibia. If the knee joint is freed, full attention should be given to strengthening thigh muscles and lengthening knee flexors and fastus intermedius. When the boot is finally removed, walking may have to some degree strengthened the foot and leg muscles; nevertheless, they will require a period of treatment before full strength and elasticity are restored.

The most frequent mistake after removal of a walking plaster is immediate return to weight-bearing, with or without crutches. A period of rest, with exercises to strengthen leg and foot muscles and lengthen peroneals and soleus muscles, should precede the period of final mobilization.

Acute muscle strain of the calf muscles occurs mostly in athletics (running, tennis, etc.) and is found mainly in the gastrocnemius. There is sometimes tear of the plantaris longus.

Raising the heel with heel pads helps the patient to walk sooner.

The following exercises emphasize resumption of normal gastrocnemius length. They are performed with the help of surface anesthetics and are done at home on a scattered basis.

1. Supine. Flexion and extension of the ankle.
   a. Pillow under knee.
   b. Knee fully extended.
2. Sitting, knee over edge of table. Flexion and extension of ankle.
3. Resistance to extension in exercises 1 and 2—given to obtain reflex relaxation of calf muscles.

Supportive prescriptions include, first surface anesthetics and rest; later, if necessary, deep heat, passive stretching and strengthening with the following exercises:

4. Add resistance to plantar flexion.
5. Standing. Hold edge of table. Rise on toes, return to starting position.
6. Standing. Hold edge of table. Place forefoot on book, heels touch floor for calf muscle stretch.
7. Step forward with injured foot, bend knee and ankle keeping heel on ground (soleus and tibialis posticus stretch).
8. Standing. Hold edge of table. Knees straight, heels on ground. Flex ankles, bringing whole body forward to stretch calf muscles.

The Ankle and Foot
Fracture of the Ankle

Severe cases, with fracture of ankle and displacement of the talus, require closed or open reduction and fixation (either internal or external).

Early mobilization of the ankle joint is possible in cases of internal fixation. Maintaining toe motion and strength and elasticity of thigh muscles should comprise the program during fixation. The period of mobilization of the ankle joint proper should always start with non-weight-bearing, scattered exercises for flexion-extension of the ankle in supine position. Strengthening the anterior tibial muscle and the extensors of the ankle, lengthening the peroneals and soleus muscle are the concerns in fractures of the ankle, whether bi-malleolar or simple fractures of the lateral malleolus.

It is imperative to avoid walking as long as the muscles are not ready for the job. Bony union precedes this period of muscular fitness, and the most common cause of prolonged disability after fracture of the ankle is premature walking or premature prolonged weight-bearing.

Time will be gained by following a program of quickly increasing resistance and weight-lifting exercises. Do not give exercises without resistance and without weight-lifting and, at the same time, allow too early walking. The last is a very common mistake and a serious one, often leading to prolonged disability, peroneal spasm, post-traumatic flat feet, etc.

One frequently finds tenderness of soleus in the lower portion if there has been walking beyond functional capacity of the foot. Sinusodial current, ethyl chloride spray and gentle deep kneading massage should be used.

Sprain of the Ankle Joint

Sprain of the ankle joint may affect both the upper and lower ankle joint and the joints of the foot. Acute sprains should be treated with surface anesthetics and immediate exercises. In more severe cases weight-bearing should be stopped. Only when surface anesthetics do not give any relief and the exercises do not seem to limber the joint or relieve pain, should immobilization be considered.

Differential diagnosis between major ligament tears and tear of Achilles tendon is essential to avoid permanent disability.

In a lesion of this joint the advantages of surface anesthetics are especially obvious, since surface anesthetics do not mask major lesion and bone damage. The joint can be treated with active motion, without weight-bearing, and there need be no fear of aggravating the condition if the "ethyl chloride test" is positive; that is, if relief follows the treatment with surface anesthetics.

The following exercises are given without weight-bearing and with relative rest in more severe cases:

1. Sitting on table. Flex and extend ankle.
2. Sitting on table. Supinate and pronate ankle.
3. Sitting on table with flexed knee. Stretch ankle. Relax. (For soleus stretch.)

In milder cases immediate weight-bearing and return to normal activities (depending on their nature) may be allowed. These additional exercises should be given:

4. Toe standing. First on floor, later with forefoot resting on a book. (For heel cord stretch, Fig. 75).
5. Standing. Supinate.
6. Standing, injured foot one step forward, knee flexed, heel firm on floor. Push knee as far forward as possible without lifting heel.

If treated within the first 24 or 48 hours, a mild sprain of the ankle should be considerably relieved, and normal work may be resumed at once. In more severe cases disability may last longer and in very severe cases may be protracted. Swelling is not a contra-indication but another urgent indication for treatment.

Sprains of the foot joints are often combined with strains of the extensor brevis of the toes. These exercises should be given after administering surface anesthetics to the region involved:

1. Sit on table, with legs dangling over edge. Flex toes. Extend and fan out. (Flexion is prescribed to provide contrast Fig. 76).
2. Standing. Flex and extend toes.

In case of major tear of the tibio-fibular ligament, or tear of deltoid ligament, operative repair is often necessary. An at-

172   *Therapeutic Exercise*

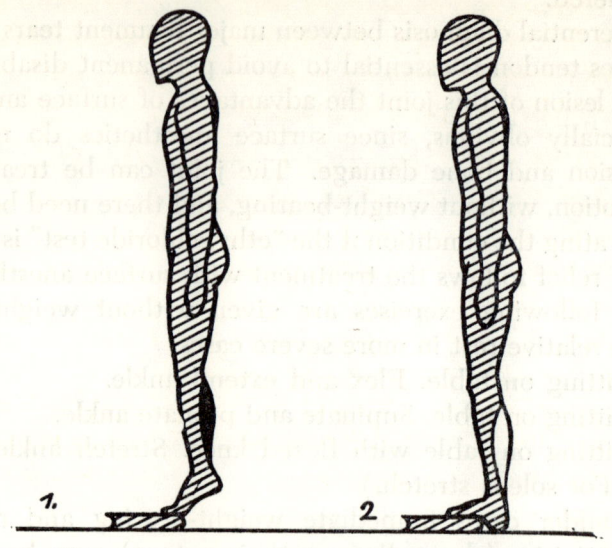

TOE STAND ON BOOK

Fig. 75

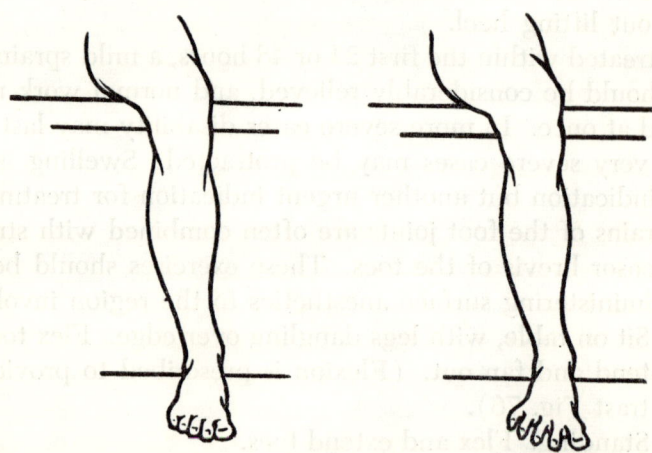

TOE SPREAD

Fig. 76

tempt at keeping the uninvolved part of the extremity near normal active motion, without weight-bearing exercises, is advisable for the ankle joint as soon as surgically possible, with resistance given, especially to strengthen dorsiflexion.

FRACTURE OF THE SHORT BONES OF THE FOOT

Fracture of the Short Bones of the Foot may often be mobilized immediately. We have found immediate mobilization after fracture of the calcaneus more satisfactory in most cases than surgical procedure or immobilization in plaster cast.

Fracture of the Metatarsal Bones and Toes: The immediate problem is to avoid aggravating present foot weakness and deformity. Weight-bearing should be postponed until it can be done without limping. Rehabilitation should stress strengthening the short foot muscles, maintaining peroneal and posterior-tibial as well as soleus length and strengthening the anterior tibial.

Chronic Foot Complaints

In infants: Early treatment by plasters, braces, and exercises can often prevent later deformities.

In young persons: A moderate degree of relaxation of the arch is very common in children and adolescents and is often not associated with muscular deficiencies or any symptoms.

If the anterior tibial muscles and the short foot muscles, especially the interossei, seem weak, the foot should be dorsiflexed against resistance or with increased weights attached to strengthen these muscles.

More severe cases may be accompanied by pronation of the heels and may require strengthening of supinators—anterior tibial muscles—and short foot muscles. If the foot's gripping ability is good, the usual exercise of picking up marbles is unnecessary, and exercises should be mainly devoted to overcoming the deficiencies present, such as weakness of dorsiflexors (*Exercise:* Sit with leg over edge of table. Dorsiflex ankle against resistance or weight; also do this exercise with foot in supination for anterior tibial strength) and of supinators (*Exercise:* Sit, feet on table, straight knees. Supinate. Same with flexed knees. Same with resistance against supination.)

At this stage contractures are not very frequent but should be watched for. If strengthening of calf muscle and soleus is prescribed by way of toe standing, it should be done on a book or box. The heel should be placed down below the edge of the box after each toe stand, in order to add a lengthening exercise to the strengthening one.

In severe cases requiring operation, the main pre-operative aim will be to obtain good muscular strength of leg and foot muscles, with special care to the anterior tibial muscle:
1. Dorsiflex foot in supination against resistance.
2. Dorsiflex foot in supination with increasing weights attached (Fig. 77).

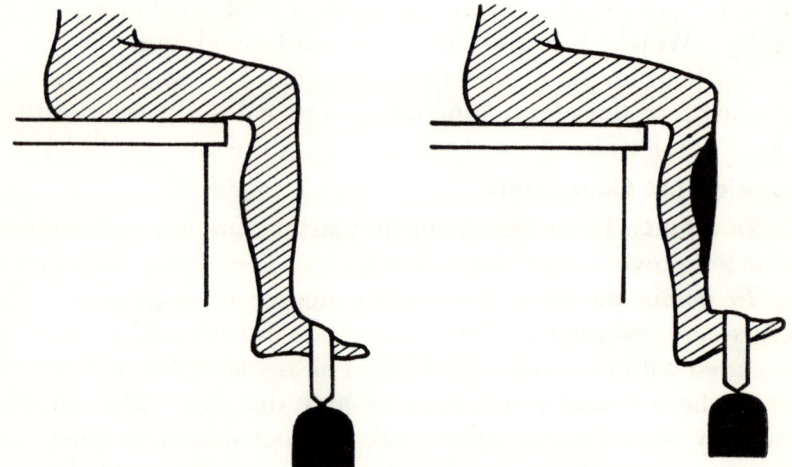

STRENGTHENING ANTERIOR TIBIAL
DORSIFLEXION – IN SUPINATION
WITH WEIGHT ATTACHED

Fig. 77

Post-operatively there should be work on maintaining the length of the peroneals, gastrocnemius and soleus, as well as on the length of the long toe flexors. Strengthening all the foot muscles, as well as the anterior tibial muscle, should be an integral part of the program. Post-operatively and after immobilization in plaster boots a scattered program (Exercises 1 and 2 above) may be indicated, and gradually increased in the usual way to full-length periods.

In older age groups: In adults, flat feet require particularly careful analysis as to contractures, painful muscle spasm and weakness. If a great number of deficient feet are examined with these points in mind, various types can be grouped together:

Type A—Soleus, gastrocnemius and posterior tibials are foreshortened, and the anterior tibials and extensors of the foot are relatively weak.

Type B—Spasm and/or contracture of the peroneal muscles are the main feature.

Type C—Contracture of the interossei is present, and the long toe flexors are contractured.

Type D—Mainly affected is the basal phalanx of the big toe. (Hallux valgus osteoarthritis of the basal toe joint, and contracture of the big toe.)

All chronic conditions occasionally produce acute and very painful foot trouble, accompanied by spasm of the overstretched muscles and local swelling of the foot, leg or mainly affected joints, or all of these combined. When these cases are acute, treatment should consist of rest, along with relief measures for acute pain, such as hot packs or surface anesthetics, followed by scattered dosage of mobilizing exercises, depending on what muscles are affected:

Type A: Dorsiflexion of foot (1) Supine, knee straight, (2) Sitting, knee flexed over pillow or edge of table, (3) Add resistance, (4) Add passive stretch, (5) Add increasing weights (Fig. 77).

Type B: Supination of foot: (1) with resistance, (2) with passive stretching.

Type C: (1) with extension of toes, with fanning out of toes (Fig. 76).

Type D: Same as for Type C.

Later, massage and manipulation of the metatarsal and toe joints may be added, and still later, or sometimes simultaneously, passive stretching supported by deep heat.

All these measures must be accompanied by sufficiently long periods of rest, with gradual return to full weightbearing activities, proper footwear and, if necessary, arch supports and metatarsal pads. In foreshortened first metatarsal (Morton toe) supports are helpful.

A proper shoe should be snug around the heel, have a straight inner contour and be wide enough and high enough in the toe to allow free movement of all toes. The heel should be wide enough to give good support, even in women's shoes: the spike heel with a minute base is conducive to recurrent and constant foot trouble. So are the swaying, unsupported strap heels on women's shoes, and tight, pointed toes in both men's and women's footwear.

It is useless to expect good results from any foot treatment unless the basis—a good shoe—has been prescribed and worn. Unfortunately, a battle with both patients and shoemakers, and frequently a losing battle, has to be fought. Women will rarely give up wearing high heels: a compromise may consist of allowing high heels for special occasions and healthy footwear for everyday.

It is a vital part of all foot treatment to convince the patient to wear proper shoes, and it should be a matter of principle not to start treatment before appropriate shoes are secured. If a patient cannot be induced to conform to this part of the supportive prescription, treatment may sometimes be rendered for relief of acute trouble, but further treatment should be refused.

The foot is by nature a gripping organ like the hand. The movement of all the toes should accompany every step, trying to grasp unevenness in the ground and thereby, with varying positions of the foot, toes and leg, produce constantly changing angles and a changing use of the various short and long muscles of foot and leg. In a city, however, this normal use of the foot does not exist and, encased in tight, inflexible shoes, treading on plane, hard pavements, the feet have gradually degenerated from supple, gripping organs to rigid inflexible parts of our lower extremity—used more like hoofs than hands. This misuse and chronic strain is the cause of many foot deficiencies in adults and must be fully understood if there is to be success in treatment and in supportive prescription.

RECOMMENDED READING

ABRAMSON, ARTHUR R.: The rehabilitation of the arthrotomised knee. *Am. J. Phys. Med.*, 32:No. 2, April 1, 1953.

Billig-Loewendahl, Evelyn: Mobilization of the Human Body. Los Angeles, Calif. The Billig Clinic.

Covalt, Donald A.: *Rehabilitation in Industry.* New York, Grune & Stratton, 1958.

Deaver, G. G. and Bown, M. E.: Challenge of crutches: prescribing crutch gaits for orthopedic disabilities. *Arch. Phys. Med.*, 26:747-758, Dec. 1945.

——————————: Challenge of crutches; crutch walking; muscular demands and preparation. *Arch. Phys. Med.*, 26:515-525, August, 1945. Correction 26:598, Sept., 1945.

——————————: Challenge of crutches; standard crutch gaits and how to keep them. *Arch. Phys. Med.*, 26:575-582, Sept., 1945.

——————————: Challenge of crutches; living with crutches and canes. *Arch. Phys. Med.*, 27:683-703, Nov., 1946.

——————————: Challenge of crutches; methods of crutch management. *Arch. Phys. Med.*, 26:397-403, July, 1945.

——————————: Challenge of crutches; daily activities on crutches. *Arch. Phys. Med.*, 27:141-157, March, 1946.

Dehne, Ernest, Schubert, James J.: Treatment of acutely compressed vertebrael body by immediate progressive mobilization. *U. S. Armed Forces M. J.*, IX:No. 12, Dec. 1958; *Mod. Medicine*, p. 164, March 15, 1959.

De Lorme, Thomas L. and Watkins, Arthur: Progressive Resistance Exercises. New York, Appleton Century Crofts, Inc., 1951.

Gaston, Sawnie R.: Low back pain due to other than intervertebral disc injuries. In Mclaughlin, H. L., *Trauma.* Philadelphia and London, W. B. Saunders Co., 1959, pp. 618-638.

——————————, and Schlesinger, Ed. B.: The low back syndrome. *Surg. Clin. of North America*, 31:2, April, 1951.

Ghormley, Ralph K.: Etiologic study of back pain. *Radiology* 70:649-653, p. 185, May, 1958.

Joseph, J.: Man's Posture. *Electromyographic Studies.* Springfield, Thomas, 1960.

Kendall, H. O., Kendall, F. P. and Boynton, D. A.: *Posture and Pain.* London, Bailliere, Tindal & Cox.

Klapp, Rudolph: *Funktionelle Behandlung der Skoliose.* Jena, G. Fischer, 1907.

Kraus, Hans: Diagnosis and treatment of low back pain. *GP*, 5:No. 4, April, 1952.

——————————: Evaluation and treatment of muscle function in athletic injuries. *Am. J. Surg.*, 98:No. 3, Sept., 1959.

——————————: Prevention and treatment of ski injuries. *J.A.M.A.*, 169:1414-1439, March 28, 1959.

——————————: Prevention of low back pain. *J. A. Phys. & Ment. Rehab.*, 6:No. 1, Sept-Oct., 1952.

———————————: The use of surface anesthesia in the treatment of painful motion. *J.A.M.A.*, *116*:2582, June 7, 1941.

KRAUS, HANS, MAHONEY, JESSE W. AND WEBER, SONYA: Immediate mobilization of certain ligamentous injuries of the knee. Pub. by the American Academy of General Practice, *GP*, *24*:No. 4, Oct. 1961. Dept. of Physical Medicine and Rehabilitation, New York University.

KRAUS, HANS AND RAAB, W.: *Hypokinetic Disease: Diseases Produced by Lack of Exercise*. Springfield, Thomas, 1961.

KRUSEN, EDWARD M.: Acute injuries to the neck. *Mod. Med.*, pp. 200-204, Sept. 15, 1960.

———————————: Pain in the neck and shoulder; common causes and response to therapy. *J.A.M.A.*, *159*:No. 13, 1282-1285, Nov. 6, 1955.

LERICHE, RENE: Qu'est-ce qu'une entrose? *Gaz. d. Hop.*, 107-325, March 7, 1934.

LOWMAN, EDWARD: *Arthritis*. Boston & Toronto, Little, Brown & Co., 1959.

McLAUGHLIN, HARRISON L.: Lesions of the musculotendinous cuff of the shoulder. Differential diagnosis of rupture. *J.A.M.A.*, *128*:563-568, June 23, 1945.

———————————: *Trauma*. Philadelphia & London, W. B. Saunders Co., 1959.

NEER, CHARLES S.: Injuries of ankle joint evaluation. *Connecticut M. J.*, *17*: 580-583, July, 1953.

SCHULTZ, WARD M.: Rehabilitation of the lower extremity amputee in a large general hospital. *New York State J. M.*, *50*:No. 17, Part 1, Sept. 1950.

SLEIGHT, R. B.: Human engineering. *Research & Engineering*, Feb., 1956.

SNOW, WILLIAM B. AND KRAUS, HANS: Novocaine iotophoresis for painful limitation of motion. *Mil. Surgeon* 95:No. 5, Nov., 1944.

STIMSON, BARBARA B.: The low back problem. *Psychosomatic Med.*, 9:210, May-June 1947.

———————————: *A Manual of Fractures and Dislocations*. Philadelphia, Lea & Febiger, 1939.

Chapter 8

THE NERVOUS SYSTEM
GENERAL INDICATIONS AND TECHNIQUE FOR THERAPEUTIC EXERCISES

TREATMENT WILL depend on the seat of the lesion and resulting disability. It is possible to differentiate main case groups depending on whether the lesion affects the lower motor neuron, upper motor neuron, the higher motor centers or proprioceptive path.

The group in which the *lower motor arc* is affected will show mainly flaccid paralysis or muscle weakness, painful muscle spasm in cases of acute irritation and, in later stages, the consequences of this painful muscle spasm, such as contracture of painful spastic antagonists or by gravity will raise another problem.

In this case group relief of pain and painful muscle spasm will be the first objective. Strengthening of weak muscle groups and returning of elasticity will follow.

While in many aspects the treatment of lesions of the lower motor neuron corresponds with exercises for musculo-skeletal conditions, there are many differences. The distribution of muscle weakness in connection with nerve injuries is often unlike that in musculo-skeletal truma. Often, also, the degree of weakness is much more pronounced in neurological conditions and will need to be rated on a considerably lower level. Frequently weakness is so severe that muscle contraction by normal nerve impulses is impossible, and electrical stimulation will be necessary to produce contraction. The use of electrical stimulation is an important addition to volitional, active exercises, with the aim of tiding a muscle over a period in which normal nerve impulses are ineffective and degeneration is likely to occur unless sufficient "artificial" exercise is provided by electric current.

The mass, the *weight*, of a muscle can be preserved to a degree by deep kneading massage. The importance of both electrical stimulation and massage for weak (0, 1 and 2) muscles has been demonstrated by experiment. Some of these findings seem to indicate that stimulation of a denervated muscle by an electric current preserves muscle excitability and that massage preserves weight or volume. However this is still controversial.

The very low muscle strength common in nerve lesions, from complete paralysis to other low grades, makes assistive exercises necessary in many cases. When larger body regions have been affected, the buoyancy of water (tank, underwater exercises) should be utilized.

Elasticity in cases of injury to the lower motor neuron can be affected in various ways. Painful muscle spasm may be present if a state of irritability exists. The generally accepted method for relief of pain is heat in the form of hot packs or hot baths. If spasm is not relieved and if the patient is not exercised and properly positioned in time, contracture may follow. In certain instances, this may, to some extent, be unavoidable. The ensuing contracture may require all forms of muscle lengthening, from reflex stretching in the beginning through strong passive stretch.

Lesion, injuries of the *upper motor neuron* or higher motor centers, result in quite another kind of motor disability, and require a different approach. In some cases these higher centers may themselves be impaired. Common to this whole group is the fact that the lower motor neuron is more or less intact and responds to stimulation of the low reflex arc—the reflex reaction will even be accentuated. It is possible to obtain movements within the normal patterns via this lower arc.

Lack of muscle strength may be present in some of the affected muscles in which volitional action cannot produce contraction. Contraction may on occasion be produced by peripheral reflexes. The use of these sometimes abnormal reflexes ("confusion") may be a valuable approach in reeducating muscles that cannot otherwise be reached.

Elasticity is frequently interfered with by spasticity. Spasticity has been previously described as a condition in which a muscle does not relax when contraction of its antagonist calls for relaxation. The spastic muscles react with contraction to every initiated movement. These muscles must be treated primarily by relaxation, which may be active or passive, but the various techniques of relaxation should always aim at ability of a muscle to relax for a purposeful movement. Lasting spasticity frequently leads to contracture that must be stretched, and may result in a need for splints and braces. Pain-relieving agents of any kind are of little use in relieving spasticity, in significant distinction from painful muscle spasm. Tetanizing current may help to relieve spasticity temporarily while fatiguing muscle groups.

Poor co-ordination is often found in upper motor neuron lesions. With certain types of brain injury, poor co-ordination may be due to a combination of reduced muscle power and spasticity. In other cases power and elasticity may be perfect, or satisfactory, but primary co-ordination may be impaired. In the first type, it will be necessary to try for improved muscle strength and relaxation. For the second, characterized by primary impairment of co-ordination, "accomplishment" exercises should be given. Co-ordinated movements should be prescribed, in increasing degrees of difficulty; better co-ordination will gradually be obtained in the same manner as skills are taught.

Another factor calling for special attention in the treatment of upper motor neuron lesions is the combination, with pathology, of other cortical or subcortical areas. Hearing, sight, speech centers and mental faculties may be affected. All these complications require special attention.

LOWER MOTOR NEURON LESION
General Aspects

The basis for prescription of exercises, as in most cases, is the muscle chart. This chart should indicate the affected muscles and the degree to which power has been diminished or the degree of contracture or spasm present. If necessary, the latter may be determined by measuring the restriction of joint motion. It should be kept in mind that these detailed charts are approximations only. They do not or cannot indicate precisely what muscles are affected, and they should be accepted for what they are — reasonably accurate indications of where muscle power is lacking. The same is true of limitation of motion due to spasm or contracture.

Muscle strength in this field is most usually graded by following the scale from zero to 5 (*see* Fig. 80); zero indicating the complete absence of muscle contracture and 5 indicating normal strength. It is a valuable and highly important basis for exercises, but, especially when children are tested, it approaches good guessing rather than accurate reckoning. These muscle tests, however, offer a sufficient basis for exercise prescription. If interpreted with a degree of caution, they are most satisfactory. When more reliable and accurate data are required for long-range prognosis, electric muscle testing may be necessary.

In lesions of the lower motor neuron difinite individual muscles are affected. The weakness of the extremities is often not as generalized as in muscular-skeletal injury in which the weakness more frequently affects muscle groups of the whole extremity. However this weakness of individual muscle groups may be distributed over large regions or over the whole body and total extremities might be affected.

In lower motor lesions affected muscles are often extremely weak, rating from zero to poor, fair or "good at best"—"good" represents a muscle that can take gravity and some resistance or weight. The treatment of "good" or fair muscles with an aim to bring them to normal is only part of the problem. In the pervious chapter we have mostly been dealing with muscles that by standards of lower motor neuron lesions would rate as in the "good" category. The treatment is concerned essentially with returning these "good" muscles to full normal strength.

These two differences, that is, the existence of more localized and of more marked weakness, require a different approach for strength building exercises. In order to do justice to the localized distribution of weakness, the exercises must be given with an aim to select the affected individual muscles often more selectively than in orthopedic problems. For example, after a fracture with weakness of elbow flexion exercise may simply be flexion of the elbow with or without resistance depending on the degree of weakness. In lower motor neuron lesion producing a selective weakness of biceps but leaving a strong brachioradialis and brachial muscle, special care will have to be taken to have this flexion of the elbow done in supination in order to avoid substitution of the affected muscles by the unaffected muscle.

Since the weakness is usually so much more marked in lower motor neuron lesion than it is in orthopedic conditions, assistive exercises, the use of underwater exercises and non-gravity exercises will be much more frequent in this type of work. When testing or exercising a muscle it is essential to stabilize its origin. If this is not done, reverse action may ensue (i.e. flexion of the pelvis on the thigh instead of thigh on pelvis when testing strength of hip flexors).

It is to be understood that the differences described above do not always prevail. There are orthopedic conditions requiring selective muscle strengthening (such as strengthening of the anterior tibial muscle in flat feet). On the other hand, "group strengthening" or strengthening of total extremities may often be required in lower motor neuron lesions or may form part of the treatment program.

As long as hope for recovery is present treatment should extend to the very weak and zero muscles. In chronic cases, or cases that have had sufficient exercise treatment, it is useless to continue working with muscles of which no practical function can be expected. It is useless to spend many hours to improve a poor muscle to a poor plus unless it can actually be returned to functional use as may be the case in finger muscles.

In children exercises will have to continue, even with low grade muscles, for years, until the growing period is over.

Peripheral Nerves

Several examples follow of typical peripheral nerve lesions which may serve as patterns for treatment of other less common cases.

Injury to the Axillary Nerve

The main symptom is impairment of abduction strength to 90°, owing to paralysis of the deltoid muscle. After treatment of the basic pathology (nerve suture, removal of a tumor, treatment of dislocation of the humerus, fracture, etc.), the arm should be kept in slight abduction to prevent overstretching of the paralyzed muscle. Motor point stimulation and massage to the muscle should be given as accessory, supportive treatment, and the following assistive exercises should be started:

1. Supine. Physiotherapist holds arm at elbow and wrist, elbow flexed, assist moving completely up to 90° abduction. Make this movement in both slight inward rotation and slight outward rotation to work all parts of the deltoid.
2. Supine. Hand on chest, arm abducted to 90°. Patient attempts to hold this position against downward pressure of therapist at elbow.
3. Standing. Hand on chest, abduct arm to 90°.
4. Standing. Touch back with fist, touch neck with fist (exercise to preserve full range of shoulder motion).

In isolated deltoid muscle paralysis, contracture of the shoulder joint can be avoided by repeating Exercise 4 several times a day for one or two minutes at a time, if necessary with assistance.

If no volitional contraction of the affected muscle is possible, massage of this muscle and motor point stimulation should be given daily.

Exercises should also be given to preserve full function in hand and elbow.

Radial Nerve Paralysis

The etiology may be pressure by callus of broken humerus, pressure of crutches (crutch paralysis) or a hard surface during sleep (Saturday night paralysis). The main symptoms, depending on the seat of injury, are wrist drop and, less frequently, paralysis of the triceps. Overstretching the extensors of the wrist should be avoided by the use of a cock-up splint. If the muscle rate is zero to 2, massage and motor point stimulation are indicated, as are passive movements of the wrist and fingers through the full range, as follows:

1. Place hand and wrist on table. Pronate. Supinate.
2. Place hand and forearm on table on ulnar side, attempt dorsi-flexion of wrist—sliding on the table to eliminate gravity.
3. Hold hand over edge of table, keep wrist extended against gravity—resistance, if possible.
4. Drop hand and wrist over edge of table. Extend wrist.
5. Place arm on table so that shoulder and elbow rest at approximately the same level—elbow is flexed—extend elbow by sliding on the table.

The Nervous System

6. Stand. Hand touches shoulder—therapist opposes extension of elbow.

Up to grade 2 muscle strength, exercises should be mainly assistive and those described above, eliminating gravity.

If contractures are present, as in older cases, passive stretching will be necessary. Use of splints to avoid or control contractures are part of the management.

The same principles apply to paralysis of the ulnar and medial nerves.

Bell's Palsy

This is the name given to paralysis of the facial nerve, with unknown etiology. Known causes for paralysis of the seventh nerve are possible conditions of the ear or the parotic gland; tumors and trauma may also be responsible. The symptoms are inability to wrinkle the forehead, close the eyelid, wrinkle the nose or move the lip on the side of the affected part. If both sides are affected, the face may become completely incapable of motion.

Treatment is by massage and galvanic motor point stimulation, preferably preceded by the use of radiant heat to make the electric stimulation less tedious. The following mirror exercises should be given as soon as the slightest motion can be elicited:

1. Wrinkle forehead. Relax.
2. Pull up eyebrows. Relax.
3. Close eyes slowly and tightly. Open slowly very wide.
4. Wrinkle nose. Relax.
5. Suck in cheeks. Relax.
6. Smile with a wide mouth. Make a small mouth.
7. Show teeth. Close mouth.
8. Thrust upper lip forward. Relax. Thrust lower lip forward. Relax.
9. Pucker chin. Relax.
10. Recite vowels a-e-i-o-u very slowly and distinctly with precise and careful lip movements.

These exercises should be done at least once, preferably four or five times, a day. In severe cases scattered dosage is advisable. In milder cases, less frequent but longer exercise periods are undertaken, to produce the impaired motion as described above.

Treatment should be continued until either full recovery has been reached or no further progress has been made in a full month of treatment. Effectiveness of any treatment of Bell's Palsy is questionable but frequently active therapy is demanded by patient and affords at least moral support in a distressing situation.

Lesions to Peripheral Nerve of the Lower Extremity

These lesions raise a different problem on account of locomotion and weight-bearing. Quite frequently braces will be necessary.

Lesion of the sciatic nerve results in paralysis of the outward rotators of the hip, flexors of the knee and all muscles from the knee down, accompanied by sensory changes. If severe enough, complete disability results, and the aid of crutches or long leg braces is required. If recovery is to be expected within a reasonably short period (a certain number of months), it will be important to stress muscle training rather than early use of the extremity in walking. If ambulation is emphasized too soon, bad walking habits may interfere with proper exercises. A compromise is sometimes necessary as to what course of treatment is taken.

Massage and motor point stimulation are essential as long as muscles are below 3, and exercises require full passive movement in the early stages in order to maintain motion for all joints. Once some muscles are up to 3 or above, exercises without weight-bearing, if possible underwater exercises, should be started. Example: A case of complete paralysis of the sciatic nerve in which hip and thigh muscles gradually return to fair but all muscles below the knee remain poor permanently. These muscles will be given electric stimulation until hope of return is gone. The whole extremity ought to be given massage of the stimulating type and the whole extremity taken through full passive range of all joints at least once a day to prevent contractures. As soon as the muscles of the thigh and hip recover enough to perform assisted movements, the following exercises should be started:

1. Lie on side, affected leg on a sliding board, (A polished board that can be used to support weak extremities by sliding movement), flex and extend knee.
2. Supine, legs straight and slightly apart, turn in toes until

they touch, then turn out until side of foot touches table.
3. Supine, slide thighs apart, bring together again.
4. Supine, legs hanging over edge of bed, try to turn in thighs raising the legs sideways.
5. Supine, bend knee, sliding foot on sheet or sliding board until the heel touches buttocks.
6. On stomach, bend knee until heel touches buttocks.

The muscles that can contract even without producing any motion have been trained to contract during the above period. But once it has been determined that the paralysis of certain parts of the extremities (in our case all the muscles below the knee) is permanent, the exercises concentrate on the returning muscles, and exercises for the unaffected muscles are added in order to get the most out of this exremity. As the fair muscles improve to good, gentle resistance is given and increased as rapidly as possible. Resistance may be increased daily to keep close to but below fatigue limits and to give sufficient manual resistance, weight exercises can be started, thus saving time for the therapist.

Leg and foot should be kept in condition for the planned use of a brace, which in this case will be ankle brace with a 90° stop at the ankle. Preventing contractures by passive movement through full range of the ankle joint once daily will accomplish this. The other exercises should have started with scattered dosage as often as the therapist is able to assist and, as soon as the assistance is not necessary, hourly for five minutes by the patient himself. As the muscles grow stronger, the exercise periods will increase in time and there will be fewer of them.

Temporary use of a long leg brace may be necessary to make earlier ambulation possible, even if short leg brace or walking without aid might be the ultimate aim.

Peroneal nerve paralysis leading to foot drop and lack of toe extension and difficulty in everting the foot are occasional complications of fractures of the fibula head or direct trauma. They are treated according to the principles above, with exercises stressing dorsiflexion of the foot and toes and eversion.

Other isolated nerve lesions are less frequent; they are usually caused by injury or local pathology and, after treatment of the basic pathology, are attended to following the principles outlined above. These peripheral nerve injuries are complicated by sensory disturbance, which cannot, of course, be affected by exercises. This problem of missing afferent stimuli may make co-ordination difficult, especially in the fingers. Occupational therapy, training of eye-finger coordination, is particularly helpful in such cases.

Plexus Injuries

The most common plexus injuries are those of the brachial plexus and are due to trauma at birth or after birth. The site of the injury determines both motor and complicating sensory disturbances. Trauma after birth may result in partial or complete tear of the plexus without fractures, or may be combined with fractures of the shoulder girdle and upper extremities. The result is a partial or complete paralysis of the affected muscles.

In cases of birth injury the problem is to preserve strength in non-affected muscles and, if diagnosed early, to preserve if possible volume (by massage).

Exercises should start as soon as the injury has been diagnosed and, therefore, consist mostly of passive positioning and conditioning. They will have to be continued throughout infancy and to the end of growing period until orthopedic procedure, if necessary, is possible.

Orthopedic procedure will deal with "what is left." For this reason it is desirable to obtain maximum strength and maximum volume in all muscles of the affected extremity. It is unwise, for instance, to let the flexors of the elbow deteriorate in an effort to produce better balance with the extensors at a lower level of power. The growth of the extremity also depends on the exercises given and on the amount of muscle volume and contractility preserved.

From the beginning contracture should be avoided by passive exercises through the full range, active exercises, assistive or resistive.

The exercises will have to be selective strengthening exercises for all muscles involved, such as described for lesion of the axillary nerve or lesions of the radial nerve. They should furthermore be exercises to prevent contractures, passively or semi-passively (that is, help with the other extremity) and finally they should attempt to compensate for what cannot be restored.

In birth injury of the plexus brachialis the use of splints to avoid overstretching affected muscles is rarely indicated, because during the first year a child is most of the time lying down and is not affected by the damaging influence of gravity. If later the affected muscles have not been restored, their return is unlikely. In the first years of life, when active participation cannot be obtained, passive exercises, exercises of the conditioning type and positioning exercises should be used. If this type of injury comes up for treatment at a later age, contractures are often present and contribute to the limitation of motion and activity; they require special passive stretching.

In adults, plexus injury through trauma or local pathology demands a different approach. After dealing with the basic pathology, an abduction splint is frequently of help to relieve overstretching of the abductor muscles; in some cases, a sling may be sufficient. Zero muscles and muscles unable to contract enough to produce movement need electric motor point stimulation and massage. Assisted and resistive exercises should be started as soon as possible.

Non-affected muscles should be kept in good condition with strengthening and limbering exercises. To avoid contracture, all joints of the affected extremity should be taken through the full range at least once a day, with special emphasis on those moved by muscles rating below 3.

Muscle Dystrophies

Under this heading various types of conditions can be differentiated. Muscle *pseudo-hypertrophy* will serve as an example. This type of case is discussed together with peripheral nerve injury because the treatment has much in common with that of flaccid paralysis. With muscle pseudo-hypertrophy exercise merely retards symptoms, and represents a losing fight, but one that must be waged to relieve suffering as long as possible and to give moral support to the patient and the patient's family.

Muscle pseudo-hypertrophy is hereditary and appears often

at an early age. The affected child cannot sit up, does not crawl or move as well as is appropriate to its age; definite muscle weakness can be found in muscles of the trunk and extremities. Diagnosis is confirmed by clinical tests and by electric muscle test. As mentioned, treatment can only check deterioration, although temporary improvement may sometimes be noticed, particularly if the child has lacked care in its first few years and when exercises can therefore bring it to a level consistent with the progress of the disease. However, parents must be cautioned not to expect more than a certain degree of improvement and a subsequent standstill for a period of time—at best.

Treatment should first try to prevent deformities of the skeleton—which are very common—by proper positioning in bed, hard mattress, feet placed against a foot board and a cradle for the blanket. Prolonged sitting up should be avoided unless the spine is protected by adequate muscles or braces. Passive exercises to the full range of all joints of the affected extremities should seek primarily to avoid contractures and subsequent deformities. Passive stretching may be necessary if there are contractures. Exercises should be given daily, below fatigue limit and, as in all cases of infant and child care, the mother must be carefully instructed in all details of the exercise procedure.

If the disease starts at a later age, it is most frequently observed in the lower extremities, although it also appears in the shoulder girdle area. More often the hip muscles are involved, and a marked thickening of the gastrocnemius muscles (pseudo-hypertrophy) is common. A typical advanced case of pseudo-hypertrophy has difficulty in rising from the floor and offers a characteristic picture when the patient tries to raise his trunk with the help of his arms climbing up his own thighs. This classical example is a frustrating experience for the patient, and should not be demonstrated in wards and clinics.

Avoiding contractures should take first place; retarding muscle weakness should be attempted with exercises below fatigue. For a while, such exercises should be given once a day and carried on over a long enough period to make it possible to give the affected extremities general strength-building work, with special and repeated exercise for the affected groups.

Lesions of the Spinal Cord
Poliomyelitis

Exercises are an important part, but only a part, of the treatment of poliomyelitis as a whole. Unfortunately, this symptomatic treatment has been over-emphasized to a point where the public fails to accept the fact that only symptoms are treated.

The child-parent relationship, the adjustment of parents to possibly permanent disabilities, should have attention from the start. It is a mistake to promise more than can be assured; this opinion is borne out by the consequences of the wide publicity the disease has received and the frequent misconception to the effect that proper treatment of infantile paralysis can positively prevent disabilities. Parents must be informed at once of the real implications of the condition, and the possibility of permanent disability must be stressed even when it is only remote.

Full recovery will be easy to accept; it is the adjustment to the child's disability that will always be difficult. Whenever parents believe they may look forward to eventual recovery, they will cling to this hope; years of heartbreaking, incessant emotional distress can be avoided by a firm prognosis at the beginning. Parents should be warned not to make treatment more difficult for themselves by adding such a psychological handicap.

In the acute stage, main attention is given to relief of pain

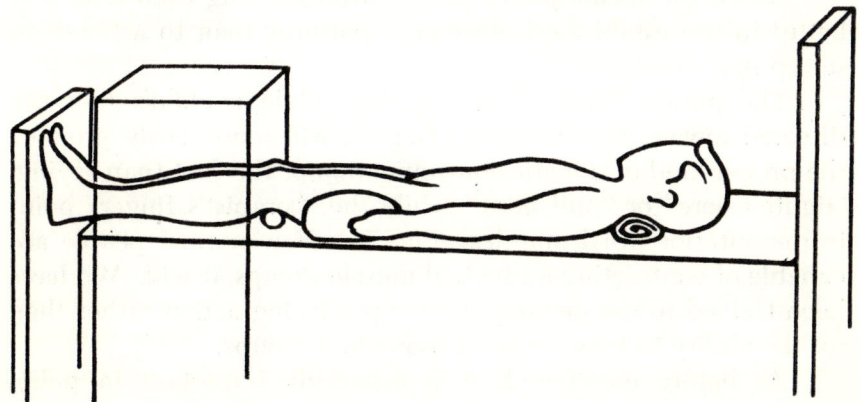

"POSITIONING" — POLIOMYELITIS

Fig. 78

and spasm and to the prevention of contractures (Fig. 78). Nevertheless, muscle strength should be preserved as much as possible from the outset. The general rule, "Watch pain limit and fatigue limit," must be most carefully adhered to. All weak muscles (for grading and charting see previous chapters and the examples that follow) should be made to work for a short time, possibly two or three times daily. The work prescribed at this acute stage should be far below the fatigue limit and should consist of guided motion, if necessary, and assisted motion through the full range possible without causing pain.

As soon as acute symptoms and pain are relieved, increase dosage. Resistance should be given to all muscles that can accept it, and anti-gravity exercises given gently to all affected, weakened muscles able to carry them out. It is a common and definite mistake to keep too far below the fatigue limit and not to give sufficient exercise value to weak muscles.

At this stage, and far into the chronic stage, stimulating massage and electric stimulation can be added to strength-building exercises. These should concentrate in the chronic stage on muscles capable of improvement. A steady increase of dosage should be maintained, and at the same time the exercise periods should be lengthened. *The most frequent mistake at the chronic stage is under-exercise.*

As for the technique of giving strengthening exercises: it is better to use established movement patterns than to attempt to set up new ones.

The phrase "touch here," spoken while a child's toes are directed toward the therapist's fingers, will more easily produce the proper kind of dorsiflexion-supination of the foot than saying, "tighten here" or "pull here," while the therapist's fingers point to the anterior tibial muscles (Fig. 79). Few normal people are capable of contracting individual muscle groups at will. We have been trained to use our muscles for producing action rather than for the ability to tense or relax individual groups.

As before mentioned, it is especially important in poliomyelitis to direct strengthening exercises to the affected muscles proper rather than to the sum total of all synergists. While it is rarely possible to pick out one isolated muscle for an exercise,

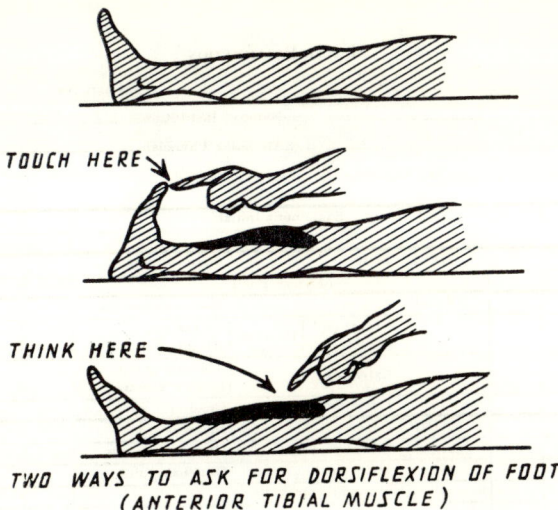

Fig. 79

this aim can be at least approximated. The muscle examination supplied by the National Foundation for Infantile Paralysis gives a good enumeration of the various movements that can be differentiated one from another (Fig. 80). *The Manual for Muscle Testing* by L. Daniels, M. Williams, and C. Worthingham gives excellent advice on how to pick out the various movements and muscles. The test movements shown in this manual can be used to advantage as a basis for the respective exercises. A muscle, for instance, that responds to the "fair" test should be made to perform this movement as an exercise. These tests are single-effort muscle tests, and when a muscle fatigues too easily to perform the test in question more than a few times in succession, it will be necessary to give it a rest while exercising other muscles and return to it for exercises after the rest period. It may be necessary also to add some exercises on the next lower testing level, if the higher test level proves too strenuous for repeated performance.

In the acute stage, muscle *spasm and pain* are the main symptoms to be dealt with. Hot baths, hot packs and certain drugs (curare, for instance) have been successfully used for this

MUSCLE EXAMINATION

Patient's Name_____ Chart No._____
Date of Birth_____ Name of Institution_____
Date of Onset_____ Attending Physician_____ M. D.
Diagnosis:

LEFT   RIGHT

					Examiner's Initials					
					Date					
					NECK	Flexors	Sternocleidomastoid				
						Extensor group					
					TRUNK	Flexors	Rectus abdominis				
						Rt. ext. obl. / Lt. int. obl. } Rotators { Lt. ext. obl. / Rt. int. obl.					
						Extensors	{ Thoracic group / Lumbar group				
						Pelvic elev.	Quadratus lumb.				
					HIP	Flexors	Iliopsoas				
						Extensors	Gluteus maximus				
						Abductors	Gluteus medius				
						Adductor group					
						External rotator group					
						Internal rotator group					
						Sartorius					
						Tensor fasciae latae					
					KNEE	Flexors	{ Biceps femoris / Inner hamstrings				
						Extensors	Quadriceps				
					ANKLE	Plantar flexors	{ Gastrocnemius / Soleus				
					FOOT	Invertors	{ Tibialis anterior / Tibialis posterior				
						Evertors	{ Peroneus brevis / Peroneus longus				
					TOES	M. P. flexors	Lumbricales				
						I. P. flexors (1st)	Flex. digit. br.				
						I. P. flexors (2nd)	Flex. digit. l.				
						M. P. extensors	{ Ext. digit. l. / Ext. digit. br.				
					HALLUX	M. P. flexor	Flex. hall. br.				
						I. P. flexor	Flex. hall. l.				
						M. P. extensor	Ext. hall. br.				
						I. P. extensor	Ext. hall. l.				

Measurements:

Cannot walk   Date   Speech
Stands   Date   Swallowing
Walks unaided   Date   Diaphragm
Walks with apparatus   Date   Intercostals

KEY

100% 5 N Normal   Complete range of motion against gravity with full resistance.   S or SS   Spasm or severe spasm.
75% 4 G Good*   Complete range of motion against gravity with some resistance.   C or CC   Contracture or severe contracture.
50% 3 F Fair*   Complete range of motion against gravity.   * Muscle spasm or contracture may limit range of mo-
25% 2 P Poor*   Complete range of motion with gravity eliminated.   tion. A question mark should be placed after the grading
10% 1 T Trace   Evidence of slight contractility. No joint motion.   of a movement that is incomplete from this cause.
0%   0 0 Zero   No evidence of contractility.

Fig. 80

purpose. Proper positioning is a further means of relieving painful muscle spasm and preventing contractures—so is splinting, etc. Once the acute stage is over, the prevention of contractures is continued and the treatment of any existing contractures should be begun.

The first and most gentle procedure is the *reflex stretch,* performed by giving resistance to the antagonist of a contractured muscle in order to bring reflex relaxation.

The next step is *active stretching,* in which the patient himself stretches a foreshortened muscle (such as a calf muscle) by forced, active pulling of the muscle through contraction of its antagonist. If necessary, passive stretching will have to be used as soon as painful spasm has subsided.

Teaching co-ordination should be reserved for the chronic stage, when it is evident that certain muscles have been permanently impaired and when, therefore, the problem of adjustment arises. From concentrating on power and elasticity as prerequisites, co-ordination quite frequently follows spontaneously after these two qualities have been restored.

Involvement of the *respiratory muscles* may be a grave complication in the acute stage of poliomyelitis. Spasm of the intercostal muscles can be recognized by their lack of movement, whereas paralysis of these muscles is identified by inverse action, that is, they bulge upon inspiration and collapse upon expiration.

Involvement of the diaphram, mainly in the direction of muscle spasm, can be seen by fluoroscopy or by clinically observing tightness and lack of motion in the epigastric region. Therapy for spasm is by application of hot packs. Breathing exercises should be started with the aim of promoting relaxation when spasm is present, and of increasing muscle action as soon as possible (*see Breathing Exercises,* p. 218). The use of the respirator will be frequently necessary.

Involvement of *throat and face muscles* and *eye muscles* most often takes the direction of loss of muscle strength and requires special attention. Artificial feeding is sometimes necessary. Swallowing, speech and breathing exercises may be needed. Exercises for the facial muscles should be the same as those described for Bell's palsy. Eye exercises ought to be given with the good eye covered and the affected eye following an object in the direction of use of the affected muscle, then with both eyes uncovered.

In all the follow-up aspects of infantile paralysis, particularly with children or adolescents, *posture* must be given special attention and posture check-ups made at regular intervals.

In order to avoid excessive repetition, the exercises in this section will be described in rather general terms, with reference to the aim rather than the specific movement. On the whole these exercises are similar to those described for lesions of the motor nerves. They will be directed to the muscles involved, avoiding substitution as much as possible.

Example: First examination of a 12 year old child on July 25th shows a number of (S) muscles in spasm, weak muscles from zero to 4. Contracture (C) can not yet be stated. Treatment consists of proper positioning, hot packs or hot baths given to muscles with spasm, muscles graded 1 and 2 are given passive assistive motion through the full range and are encouraged to contract. Muscles graded 3 and 4 are given active motion through full range once to twice a day below pain limits and far below fatigue limit. Each movement may be made two or three times only if the general condition of the child is still poor. The number of packs is gradually deceased until spasm has subsided and they are no longer necessary.

August 2nd: There is still some mild spasm in some muscles; however, in some of the previously painful muscles, spasm has subsided and mild contracture is discernible. Some of the 4 muscles have recovered to 5, some of them have deteriorated to 3, and similar changes of improvement on one side and increasing weakness of the other in other affected muscles. The exercise program should now add active reflex stretch for all C muscles (for instance, resistance to quadriceps in order to relax hamstrings). The 3 muscles should receive anti-gravity exercises; gentle resistance for the 4 muscles will be added, and 1 and 2 muscles will be exercised within the limit of their function, i.e., exercises without gravity, assistance should be given to the 2 muscles and contractions will be attempted. The exercise period should be increased in length, and two or three, if possible more, exercise periods should be arranged for.

August 10th: There is no more spasm; some muscles still show contractures. By now the tendency of some of the muscles to weaken further, and others to recover, has been established. In other words, it will be possible to determine which of the muscles tend to recover and which offer a less favorable prognosis. Treatment should omit hot packs except previous to exercise periods if contractures are severe. Stretching will be done actively as before, and gently, passively by the therapist. The zero to 2 muscles should receive motor point stimulation, all the weak regions to benefit from a stimulating massage. The exercise period may reach twenty minutes or more and three or four of these periods can be given. Resistance to the 4 muscles should increase rapidly from now on.

October 20th: Contractures have been relieved, definite patterns of muscle weakness have been established. If a muscle under the proper care has not at least reached the poor stage at this point, it will most likely have no chance of further recovery. Exercises should concentrate on muscles from 2 to 4. Passive exercises will be made to maintain joint range when zero to 1 muscles cannot provide for it. The aim will be to avoid occurrence of contractures. Exercise periods should consist of thirty minutes twice a day, and the exercises for 3 and 4 muscles should be close to, though still below, fatigue limit, increasing as quickly as tolerated.

December 20th: Braces will be prescribed if necessary. Exercises should concentrate on 3 and 4 muscles, with substitution to be started where necessary; and co-ordination exercises may now form part of the program. Muscle strengthening may further concentrate on certain groups or individual muscles, which may be important for future surgery.

Transsection of Spinal Cord

The continuity of the spinal cord may be interrupted, as a result of acute infection or injury. Functional recovery may be partial or complete, or there may be no recovery at all. Depending on the level at which the lesion occurs and depending on whether the transverse interruption is complete or partial, various parts of the body are affected. The result, as regards motor function, is mainly a spastic paralysis. The most frequent lesions are afflictions of both lower extremities.

Paraplegia

If the lesion results in permanent paralysis of both legs, the problem is mainly to enable the patient to adjust himself to the state of disability. It is important to keep the lower extremities in such a condition that wearing braces is feasible (double leg braces with a pelvic band and sometimes with a trunk brace attached). Management of the body with these double leg braces and with the help of crutches depends entirely upon the upper extremities and what remains of the trunk muscles. These remaining muscles must be strengthened as much as possible, and special stress should be laid on strengthening the extensor group, as well as the flexors, of the arms, because walking on crutches depends largely on the use of these extensor muscles.

The affected extremities show spastic paralysis and tend to develop contractures. In the rehabilitation program the extremities are kept, as far as possible, with the knees extended, ankles at 90° and hips extended. In cases of complete and permanent interruption of a cord, active exercises cannot be applied to these extremities, which must be taken through the desired joint range by passive movements, in order to keep or regain the proper position of the joint required for braces.

Exercises should begin as soon as possible from a general medical point of view for patients in whom an advanced degree of recovery, or even partial recovery, may be expected. Muscle tests will show the presence of spasticity possible contracture and weakness. These findings should be charted and the exercise program based mainly on the muscle chart.

Avoiding contractures and relieving spasticity if it can be effected should be the principal concern of treatment for a long time, as well as strengthening, where return of strength can be hoped for. Pain may be a severe complication in these cases and medication, or even surgical care, may be required. Some times triggerpoints develop in spastic muscles and can be relieved by injection.

Multiple Sclerosis

This disease, as yet of unknown origin, affects various parts of the central nervous system. Its onset is slow, but it develops to more severe stages, though temporary improvements are frequent. These periods of improvement alternate with periods of increased symptoms. Multiple sclerosis not only affects the motor neurons but is dispersed throughout the nervous system and may attack any of its area.

The symptoms are accordingly variable. Some symptoms that can benefit from exercises are: muscle weakness, occasional spasticity in certain muscle groups, contractures and poor or completely lacking co-ordination leading to awkwardness, difficulties in gait or total inability to walk.

Muscle charting should be the basis for an exercise program. Perhaps even more than in other cases, thorough muscle testing must precede an outline of treatment. Scattered dosage of exercises is necessary, because the patient is easily inclined to fatigue and to avoid damage the exercises must be done below fatigue and pain limits.

The first step is usually the stretching of existing contractures and the slow strengthening of those muscles capable of developing more strength. After these preliminaries, co-ordination should be attempted, and compensation by present muscles for those which cannot be re-educated. The patient has to learn to "get along with what he has," and it is sometimes surprising to what extent this can be achieved with proper treatment.

The physical therapist must be fully aware that, at best, only temporary relief and adjustment can be obtained. Future recurrences must be expected, which will leave the patient with diminished motor ability. It will be possible again to restore some of this by proper training, but recovery will be less than after the first occurrence and treatment.

The final purpose in the treatment of multiple sclerosis is not full recovery but regaining as much motor ability as possible under the circumstances and preserving this as far as possible. In consequence, many years of relatively good motor ability may be gained, and patients can be kept active for relatively long periods of time. Continual treatment and continually maintaining exercises is very worth while, depressing as the eventual outlook may be.

The following is an example of treatment for multiple sclerosis:

Left lower extremity mainly is affected. Balance severely impaired so that patient has to use crutches. Condition is variable and must be retested at short intervals. Patient suffers frequently from painful spasms which are treated with hot packs.

Program: (1) Breathing: As preliminary for relaxation training and to avoid straining when crutch walking. (2) Strengthening abdominal muscles and arms (Since patient has to use crutches strong trunk and upper extremities are of great importance). (3) Relaxation of hip muscles. Active relaxation with use of right lower extremity for comparison in reflex stretching. (4) Coordination for both lower extremities. (5) Active relaxation of whole body.

Exercises are to be given daily for a total of one-half to one hour, preferably distributed in two sessions. Less if not tolerated without fatigue.

Tabes Dorsalis

This disease appears at any time between five to forty years after syphilitic infection. Pathology is due to inflammatory reactions and degeneration of the dorsal funiculi of the cord and of nuclei in the brain stem.

The symptom commonly treated by exercises is "locomotor ataxia." Ataxia of the gait is among the early symptoms, together with "lightning" pains and incontinence. The ataxia of gait, which is the main object of treatment, is more pronounced in the dark when visual correction is not possible. Loss of vision is a complication, as are atrophic disturbances such as Charcot joints, hypertonia and atrophy of muscles.

Exercises are mainly directed toward improving what coordination is left in the lower extremities.* (Muscle strength and muscle elasticity do not usually require special attention.) When

---

* Frenkel has described a number of exercises of this type.

giving these co-ordination exercises, it is important to proceed gradually and not to jump too rapidly to higher levels of accomplishment. The exercises should be performed with emphasis on precision, and co-ordination should be aimed at by way of "accomplishments." There should be four stages of exercises: (1) guided; (2) unguided; (3) with help of the eyes; (4) with eyes closed if possible.

The following suggestions are offered:

A. *On back:*
   1. Bend leg at hip and knee. Slide heel on bed. Stretch leg.
   2. Bend leg halfway. Stretch.
   3. Bend both legs at hip and knee. Stretch legs.
   4. Touch left knee with right heel. Touch right knee with left heel.

B. *Sitting:*
   1. Sit down slowly without dropping into chair.
   2. Cross right ankle over left. Cross left ankle over right.
   3. Cross right knee over left. Hold legs parallel. Cross left knee over right.
   4. Get up slowly from chair.

C. *Standing:*
   1. Try to walk between two lines spaced a foot apart.
   2. Walk so that all steps are uniform in length.
   3. Balance training.
   4. Obstacle walking.

LESIONS TO UPPER MOTOR NEURON AND UPPER MOTOR CENTERS

Congenital Lesions of Upper Motor Neuron and Upper Motor Centers (Fig. 81).

Cerebral Palsies

First described by Little in 1853, these conditions have been rather neglected until the last two decades when their importance, and the possibility of treatment and improvement, has been realized. This fact is to a large extent due to the work of Winthrop Phelps.

It is now generally accepted that only a certain percentage

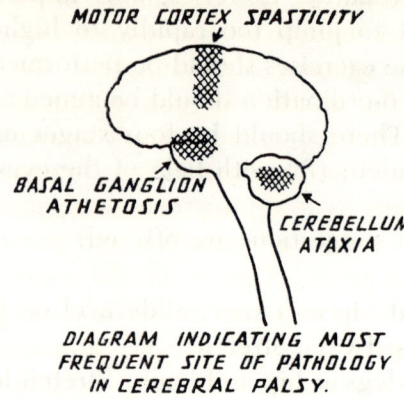

DIAGRAM INDICATING MOST FREQUENT SITE OF PATHOLOGY IN CEREBRAL PALSY.

Fig. 81

of children born with cerebral palsy are mentally deficient, and of these a still smaller percentage is not amenable to training. It is likewise agreed that cerebral palsy children have been underrated, owing to their lack of motor ability and to their inability to express themselves. Because of these failings, they have scored low in psychological tests and in some cases have been erroneously classified as mentally deficient. As motor abilities improve with training, the psychological test scores often improve, and borderline cases or even cases with relatively low I.Q.s, advance to a fairly normal rating.

All these various aspects have to be brought together, either in special institutions for treating this type of patient, or, if the treatment is carried out in general hospitals, by assuring all the specialist services involved. One fairly satisfactory solution is to co-ordinate the actual treatment procedure by arranging consultant clinics that include the staffs of the treatment clinics (occupational therapy, physical therapy, pediatrics and social service) and to make the consultant clinics reach the various decisions as to future steps.

One person should remain responsible for the patient to insure coordinated management and planning.

It has been recognized that cerebral palsy children represent not necessarily a total loss, and this fact has given rise to new and sometimes exaggerated hopes on the part of parents. Some of the people concerned in the treatment have been led to be too sanguine; and optimism has sometimes been expressed by too bright a prognosis. Unfortunately, the outlook for the cerebral palsy child is still not one of complete success; yet parents, grasping at every straw, are only too anxious to welcome any hope that is held out and are willing to expect far too much. One of the first steps in accepting a cerebral palsy child for treatment should be a complete evaluation and parents should be informed of the prospects. This is all the more important since emotional elements have come to have a disproportionate influence on treatment procedures and arrangements for these children, and they have not been found helpful to anybody concerned.

Before outlining the exercise techniques used in various types of cerebral palsy, one problem common to all should be mentioned. Since treatments are given primarily to lower age groups, they have to be carried out at home by parents, unless the child is institutionalized. Treatment should be for half an hour, six days a week, and very few clinics are now equipped to deal with patients so frequently. An important part of treatment, therefore, consists of instructions to the parents. Equally important is the solution of behavior problems in the child. Most of these children present such problems, and guidance of parents, as well as of the child, is a necessary preliminary to treatment. Those concerned must be constantly on the alert for evidence of these behavior problems.

For each case the exercise program should be based, as always, on a muscle test. It is particularly important to consider all complicating factors and to decide what is to be the immediate aim. The goal of the whole rehabilitation process ought to be defined; and both immediate and final aims will influence the shaping of the exercise program. For instance, when the immediate aim is ability to sit, the final aim ability to walk, the exercise program should first stress trunk strength and spend less time on the lower extremities. Once the immediate purpose has been accomplished, more and increased exercises should be given to the lower extremities, and trunk exercises decreased or omitted.

Muscle tests evaluate and chart deficiencies in muscle power: zero cerebral muscles, deficiencies in elasticity, spasticity, contractures, rigidity; poor co-ordination: athetoid movements, balance difficulties and ataxic symptoms.

Activities of daily living test (ADL) and accomplishment charts (see Fig. 13) complete the tests.

Tests should be repeated every one to three months, the exercise program changed according to results.

Graphs of accomplishment help register progress—they are especially significant in ataxia and athetosis.

A number of assisting devices are valuable in the treatment of cerebral palsies, some of the more important being skis, walkers, relaxation chairs and cut-out tables (see illustrations). Twisters—rubber bands attached to the soles of the shoes on one side and fixed to a belt around the waist after circling the lower extremities—are sometimes useful.

The main groups of cerebral palsies will be discussed: (1) the groups in which the preponderant problems are spasticity, (2) ataxies, and (3) the athetoses.

Spastic Paralysis. Lesion affects the upper motor neuron and results in a spastic paralysis, which may include all four extremities (spastic quadriplegia), two extremities (diplegia), if relating to both arms or both legs, and hemiplegia if affecting one arm and one leg on the same side. Monoplegia is present if only one extremity is affected. The cranial nerves are also frequently involved. The muscles of the tongue are often affected, creating speech difficulties and drooling. Muscle examination may show spasticity, contractures, weakness and poor co-ordination.

In the early age group (up to three or four years) the technique of exercises given to relieve spasticity and to increase muscle strength should be based upon conditioning exercises (see *Technique*). Reflex movements can be used. As soon as active co-operation can be obtained, active exercises should be stressed. If there is only partial involvement of one or more extremities, conditioning exercises should be confined to the involved area and not include motions that can be well done spontaneously unless desirable for coordination. By keeping the exercise program down to the most necessary requirements, more exercise value can be given.

Passive stretching will have to form part of the exercise program if contractures exist. This passive stretching should be done with special care, in order to avoid a stretch reflex and thus increase spasticity. Some authors feel that the upper extremities should not be exercised until handedness has been determined in occupational therapy, and then work should be stressed with the leading hand only. This procedure holds good especially if there are speech difficulties or a history of seizures.

Further exercises for the lower extremities are ski-walking and walking in a walker, with or without abduction board. Ski-walking (see illustration) prevents the child from raising the heel from the floor, provides a stable basis and the assistance of poles and helps from a walking pattern. However, it should not be used indiscriminately for all spastic children with afflictions of the lower extremities. Some children have a definite aversion for the skis and do well in walkers, while others have no difficulties with the ski-walker. Certain hemiplegia cases respond better and are able to walk better if treated with brace only or walker.

At later age, the exercise technique should change. While conditioning exercises may still be necessary to improve an incomplete movement pattern, it will be possible to *teach active relaxation*—this should never be neglected. Even a three or four-year-old child often co-operates more readily when a demand is made upon his mind. Continuing nursery rhymes and conditioning at later years arouses resistance from the more alert children, who resent being treated as babies. It is surprising how young children of three or four, or even younger, understand the process of active relaxation and put it to use. While active relaxation is generally used from the start in athetosis, it is, for some reason, much less commonly used for spasticity, and conditioning exercises predominate in most treatment plans.

Active or conscious relaxation should start with teaching the difference between a tensed and a relaxed muscle. Next, teach relaxing spastic muscles at rest. Later, seek for relaxation with passive movement, assistive movement, active movement without assistance, and finally resistive movement against gravity. Resistance given to the antagonist of the spastic muscle (Reflex-relaxation—*see Technique*, p. 41) is used to advantage to produce relaxation in the spastic muscle.

Strength-building exercises are necessary for weak or zero muscles. Zero cerebral muscles that cannot be strengthened by direct volitional work may be influenced by conditioning exercises or by "confusion" movements.

One of the typical disabilities in these children is lack of active dorsiflexion of the affected ankle. Nevertheless, a "confusion" movement (Fig. 82) can often bring about active dorsiflexion. If the child is placed with legs hanging from the edge of the table and is asked to lift his knee against resistance, the ankle is brought into dorsiflexion by a reflex impulse occurring when the resistive movement is performed. Such "confusion" movements can be used to strengthen and train the dorsiflexors of the ankle. Step-by-step confusion is given, first with the resistance of the therapist, later with the child providing resistance with his own hands, and still later, with the child's hand merely being placed on the thigh without giving much resistance, but with resistance "though of."

Once spontaneous "confusion" is achieved, it can be practiced while standing (Fig. 83), and from then on carried over into the walking pattern. Spasticity of the gastrocnemius and soleus groups and contractures in this group often need attention before a confusion action can result in movement and not waste itself in useless tugging at its antagonist.

Two examples follow of treatment programs in spasticity, to be regarded only as skeleton outlines of a full program:

Example A

Case—A two-year-old child with spastic quadriplegia. No speech because of tongue involvement. Lateral duction and extension is lacking in tongue motion. The main muscle findings are:

a) Upper extremities—Spasticity of adductors of arm, flexors of elbow and fingers, a weakness of wrist and finger extensors. Both sides are similarly affected, and spasticity moderately severe. Contractions: none.

b) Lower extremities—Slight spasticity of gluteal regions, outward rotators of hip, severe spasticity of adductors, gastrocnemius soleus and toe flexors, and mild spasticity

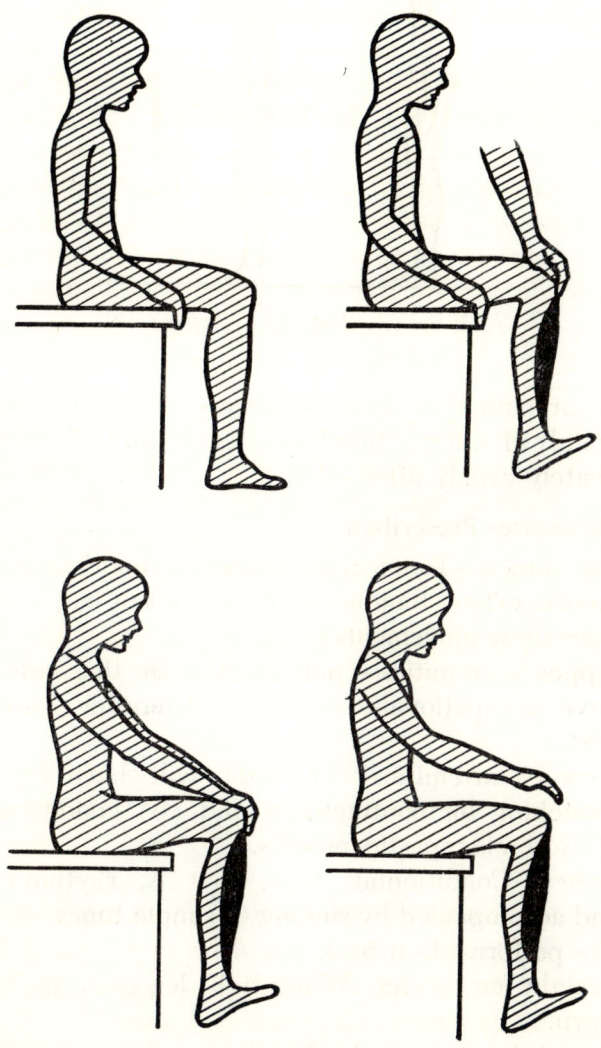

Fig. 82

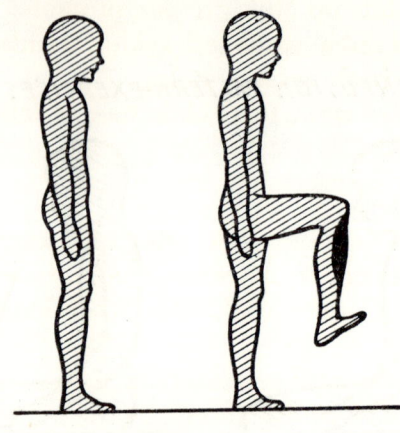

Fig. 83

of pronators of foot, weakness of ankle dorsi-flexors, mainly of anterior tibial muscles. Again both sides approximately evenly affected.

Types of Exercises Prescribed

(1) For tongue—Touch right corner of mouth, left corner of mouth, extend tongue (a lollipop or salt bag is used to induce these movements).

(2) Upper extremities—(not charted in this case) should have occupational therapy to determine leading hand first.

(3) Lower extremities—(charted) will have (a) passive stretching for contractures, and (b) conditioning exercises to relax spastic muscles.

Exercises: Conditioning type, that is, rhythmically performed and accompanied by singing of simple tunes.

All are performed on back.

1. Straight leg raising. While right leg goes up, left comes down.
2. Spread legs apart slowly, sliding them on table. Slide slowly together again.
3. Rotate straight legs inward. Outward.

The Nervous System

4. Bend right knee while right foot slides toward buttocks. While right foot slides back to straight position, left foot starts to slide up (this exercise promotes reciprocation).
5. Flex right ankle while left ankle extends. Reverse.
6. Supinate both ankles. Relax.
7. Flex toes of right foot while toes of left foot extend. Reverse.

Example B

Case—A five-year-old child with spasticity and weakness as in Example A. There is, however, contracture of adductors and of calf muscles. Cannot walk. No other handicaps.

Suggestions:
1. Teach child active relaxation.
2. Stretching of contractures.
3. Teach flexion-extension in hip and knee in lying position, as follows: (a) passively (b) actively—with assistance (c) actively—without assistance. (Aim: Local relaxation.)
4. "Confusion" with dorsiflexion.
5. Ski walking later, walker (Fig. 84).
6. Use of braces will probably be necessary.

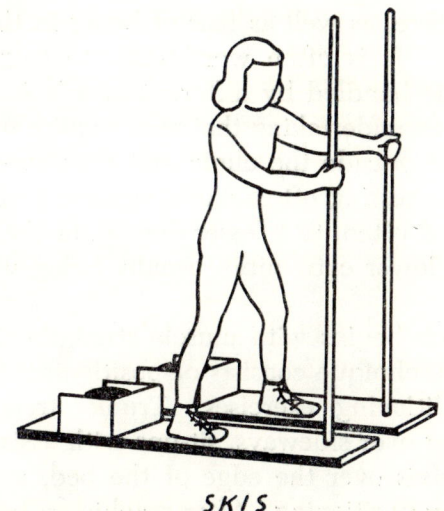

SKIS

Fig. 84

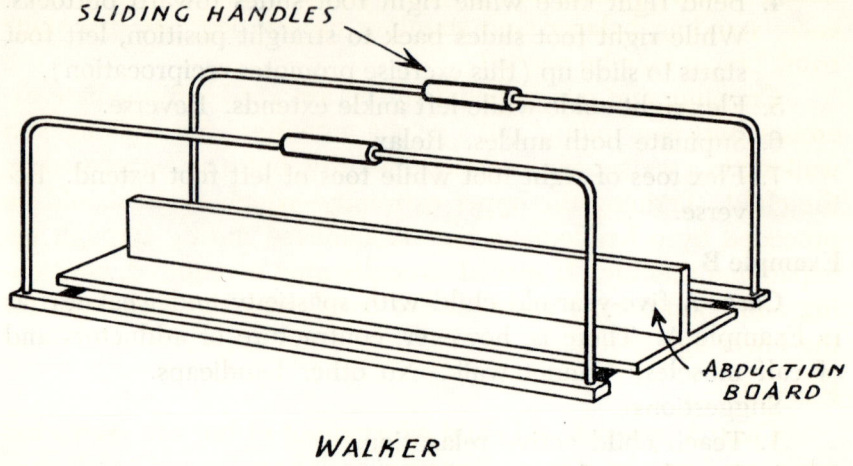

WALKER

Fig. 85

Ataxia. Lesion is usually found in the cerebellum. The basic difficulty is lack of balance and coordination, accompanied by general muscle weakness. The main motor symptoms are inability to stand, sit, keep the head raised or make well-defined movements with the extremities. Fear of heights is usually present in this clinical picture, as well as fear of being in the hands of unfamiliar persons. It is often worthwhile to suggest to parents that the child be handled by different people in order to break down this fear, an undertaking that may require weeks of preliminary adjustment outside the clinic and thus save valuable time later on. Muscle testing often shows weakness of the trunk and neck muscles and often, to a lesser degree, of the muscles of the extremities, the lower extremities usually being weaker than the upper.

The program begins with muscle strengthening. For lower age groups the technique consists of positioning exercises and, if necessary, conditioning exercises. Trunk strength should be sought by rolling over sideways, sit-ups with assistance, positioning with the pelvis over the edge of the bed, and head flexion and extension by positioning. After reaching a certain minimum of trunk strength, move on to the following accomplishments:

sitting balance (timed and graphed), head balance, kneeling balance, standing balance and standing on one leg. At this stage trunk braces may be needed.

Crawling and quadrupedal stance are good intermediate exercises between rolling and upright activities. Ski-walking and walking in a walker are sometimes helpful, but may be refused by the child. Training the upper extremity—which again should be proceded by a handedness test—is achieved mostly through occupational therapy. If special strengthening is required, positioning and conditioning exercises are once more the technique for the lower age group.

Example

Case: A two-year-old child who cannot sit but can crawl; has some quadrupedal stance. Posterior neck muscles and trunk muscles are fair; abdominals poor. Anterior neck muscles are poor.

Suggestions:
1. Trunk strengthening by positioning.
2. Attempt to get balance with trunk brace.
3. Attempt to produce neck strength.
4. Standing balance with skis.
5. Ski walking.
6. Standing balance with support.
7. Walking in a walker.
8. One leg balance, with and without support.
9. Walking without support.

Athetosis may be caused by a basal ganglion lesion. The symptoms are involuntary motions while at rest, and involuntary motions superimposed on any attempt at volitional activity. Any region of the body may be more or less severely involved. If not treated from early childhood, these patients frequently try to overcome their handicap by bracing their own joints and their muscles—by tensing the antagonists simultaneously. The result is "tension athetoid." The treatment with exercise in athetosis is based on relaxation—relaxation taken here in the widest sense, meaning the suppressing of contraction stimuli to muscles other than those intended for contraction.

Muscle tests indicate the distribution and degree of involuntary motion at rest and in various standard positions. Contractures, and their degree, must be observed in this test. Relaxation should start at rest and from the resting position in which the patient shows the least number of involuntary movements. Various other resting positions (prone, sitting, lying on side, etc.) should be used to train relaxation at rest. At the same time the usual stages of relaxation procedure must be gone through, step by step. Relaxation should be developed with passive, assisted and finally free movements.

Breathing exercises for relaxation, relaxed breathing are often basic conditions for tongue relaxation and improvement of speech. Speech problems may be aggravated by pitch deafness.

Stabilizing braces are helpful in many of these cases, obviating relaxation for the braced parts of the body.

This group of patients is often of normal, or above average mentality, and it is therefore doubly important to provide them with means of expression. The use of relaxation chairs, which make relaxation easier, and of electrical typewriters, which make writing possible when it is quite impossible by hand, are media that may be advantageous. Relaxation is not the only approach: sometimes active "splinting" produces good results.

RIGIDITY

Rigidity may be caused by diffuse hemorrhage of the brain—it is more often the result of encephalitis. Frequently it is associated with tremor.

The symptom of rigidity is lack of relaxation of the affected muscle group. These muscles, however, do not show the stretch reflex and do not show spasticity. They differ from contractures, which require much more intense stretching before they respond. Rigidity, frequently leads to contractures, and treatment of such cases consists largely in avoiding them. Since rigidity is often associated with extensive impairment of learning centers, there is often serious mental retardation.

MOTOR RETARDATIONS

With general awareness of the cerebral palsy problem, it is clear that there is an increasing number of children that do not fit into any special category of either central or peripheral motor lesion, but show retarded abilities in motor development. Sometimes these undiagnosed cases may be mild examples of the above group; sometimes they may be the result merely of slow motor development.

All these cases require special muscle testing before treatment. By positioning, reactions and muscle strength can be gauged as a whole. Involuntary motions and spasticity, as well as the symptoms of ataxia, should be looked for before the cases are classified as in the general group of "motor retardations."

The treatment technique in these cases consists of positioning and conditioning exercises, depending on what deficiency has been found and what accomplishment is sought for. Accomplishment charts and graphs are of help. When there is marked deficiency of one or more muscle qualities it is important to improve muscle function before stressing accomplishments.

POST-NATAL AND ADULT LESIONS TO THE UPPER MOTOR NEURON

The etiology in this group may be trauma to the head or inflammation of the central nervous system, due to infection such as measles, influenze (causing encephalitis), tumors, cerebral hemorrhage due to hypertension, thrombosis, etc. Persons of all ages can be affected. The motor symptoms are most frequently hemiplegias. Involvement of eye, tongue, pharynx and head muscles is not infrequent. The groups of central lesions described in foregoing sections—spastic paralysis, ataxia, athetosis and rigidity—may occur, depending on the site of lesion.

Complicating factors may be as far-reaching as those of cerebral palsy and may require the same combination of various specialists' attention. For the older patients, this inclusive approach culminates in an attempt at rehabilitation leading back to the occupation performed before the lesion was incurred. If mental capacity has not been interfered with, the whole problem will be simplified to the re-learning of lost motor abilities rather than the learning of entirely new skills. Exercises for these hemiplegias constitute only a part of the total effort needed to rehabilitate the patient.

The basic exercise problem differs in one important point from that presented by congenital cerebral palsy: all these secondary brain lesions once possessed normal motor patterns, most of the patients are older. It will, therefore, usually be possible to omit conditioning exercises as one of the techniques. The same holds true of positioning exercises. These two types of exercise may be used for very young patients but never for patients old enough to co-operate actively. In these cases group motor patterns have been established which will be of help in re-training for co-ordination. Reciprocal motion for the lower extremities will rarely be needed.

SPASTIC HEMIPLEGIA

Shortly after the cerebral accident has occurred, a flaccid stage usually precedes spastic hemiplegia. Muscle charting will, as in congenital cerebral palsies, be only part of the whole evaluation determining the exercise program. The final and immediate purposes of the program should be established or at least outlined. Treatment aids (splints and braces) should be suggested when necessary. Muscle charts will note and grade: (1) Poor elasticity—spasticity and contractures, (2) poor strength—weak, zero, cerebral muscles, and (3) poor co-ordination.

It has been found most effective to concentrate, even at this early, flaccid stage, on the prevention of contractures and spasticity rather than to attempt to produce active muscle contraction. For this reason, as assistive treatment do not use electric stimulation or any but gentle massage. Full range of motion of all affected joints is to be undertaken once or twice a day, while the patient is positioned on a flat, hard bed, with knees extended to 180° and ankles in a 90° position, preferably placed against a board. As soon as active response of the muscle recurs, and when the first signs of spasticity appear, efforts should be directed toward active relaxation, again in preference to strength-building.

Once the full picture of spasticity has developed, and zero muscles have shown up, stimulation and active exercise of the latter groups are to be added to the relaxation program, which still remains predominent.

A similar approach is made in the treatment of eye, tongue and face muscles.

When a patient gets up and starts walking, there is often an increase of spasticity of the lower extremities. It is therefore advisable to try to postpone walking, especially in young people, until the patient understands active relaxation thoroughly enough to use it in his walking pattern.

With older patients, general health and living conditions must be considered. Such patients will require earlier ambulation. The patient's mentality may make a speed-up program imperative in order to avoid invalidism as an accepted fact. For patients with a more ambitious goal, slower programs are preferable, concentrating on better relaxation and better form of movement.

The use of "confusion" movement, whenever present should be made the most of. Carry over to normal walking is frequent.

Example of a Spastic Hemiplegia

Case: 60 year old patient. Right hemiplegia occurred three months ago. High blood pressure. Able to walk with help for last six weeks. Speech difficulty—"mixes up" words—aphasia. One exercise period of one-half hour daily. Muscle chart shows: a) Upper extremity—spasticity of adductors of shoulder, flexors of elbow, wrist and fingers, contracture of flexors of wrist and fingers and weakness of finger and wrist extensors. b) Lower extremity—spasticity of outward rotators of hip, adductors and calf muscles, contracture of gastrocnemius soleus, and weakness of inward rotators of hip and anterior tibial.

Exercise Program

1. *Stretch* gastrocnemius soleus, flexors of wrist and flexors of fingers.
2. *Relax.* Upper extremity—shoulder adductors.
   elbow flexors.
   wrist flexors.
   finger flexors.
   Lower extremity—outward rotators of hip.
   adductors.
   calf muscle.
3. *Strengthen*
   Upper extremity—finger extensors.
   wrist extensors.

Lower extremity—inward rotators of hip.
　　　　　　　　　　anterior tibial (confusion).
4. *Speech*. Speech therapist.
5. Patient is given *night splint* to stretch flexors of wrist and fingers.
6. *Short leg brace* is given.

ADULT ATAXIAS

Ataxias due to post-natal lesions are approached like cerebral palsies. The pre-existence of movement patterns facilitates and hastens the procedure whenever the basic lesion is not progressive. Here too, the necessary strength, if lacking, should be restored before asking for accomplishments that otherwise are frustrating and retard development.

Several valuable techniques have been perfected by different authors (See Recommended Reading).

RECOMMENDED READING

DEAVER, GEORGE G.: Hemiplegia and rehabilitation. *Oklahoma State M. J.*, 53:9:625-628, Sept. 1960.

————————: Evaluation of disability and rehabilitation procedures of patients with spinal cord lesions. Instit. Crippled and Disabled, 1948.

FRENKEL, HENRICH S.: *The Treatment of Tabetic Ataxi by Means of Systematic Exercise; an Exposition of the Principles and Practice of Compensatory Movement.* Blankiston, Philadelphia, 1902.

HELLEBRANDT, F. E.: Physiology of motor learning as applied to the treatment of the cerebral palsy. Reprint from *Quart. Rev. Pediatrics*, 7: No. 1, Feb. 1952.

HUTCHINSON, E., LANCTOT, E. H. AND PHELPS, W. M.: *Handbook on Physical Therapy for Cerebral Palsy.* Pub. by Ohio Society for Crippled Children, Inc., Distributed by State Dept. of Education, Division Special Education, Columbus, Ohio.

KENDALL, H. O. AND KENDALL, F. P.: Orthopedic and physiotherapy objectives in poliomyolitis treatment. *Physiotherapy Rev.*, 27: No. 3, 159-165, May/June, 1947,

KENNY, ELISABETH: *Treatment of Infantile Paralysis in the Acute State.* Minneapolis, St. Paul, Bruce Publishing Co., 1941.

KNOTT, MARGARET AND VOSS, DOROTHY. Proprioceptive Neuromuscular *Facilitation.* Hoeber-Harper, 1956.

KRAUS, HANS: Treatment of cerebral palsy. *Med. Clin. North America*, May, 1948.

―――――――――――――: Therapeutic exercises in pediatrics. *M. Clin. North America*, New York, May 1947.
LOVETTE, ROBERT W.: *Treatment of Infantile Paralysis.* Philadelphia, P. Blakiston Son & Co., 1917.
MEAD, SEDGWICK, AND KNOTT, MARGARET: The use of ice in the treatment of joint resistrictions, spasticity and certain types of pain. Calif. Rehab. Center.
MERRITT, H. HOUSTON, METTLER, FRED A. AND PUTNAM, TRACY J.: *Fundamentals of Clinical Neurology.* Philadelphia & Toronto, The Blakiston Co., 1947.
PHELPS, W. M.: Progress in orthopedic surgery for 1944. Neuro-muscular disorders exclusive of poliomyolitis. *Arch. Surg.,* 51:315-318, Nov.-Dec. 1945.
―――――――――――――: Recent trends in cerebral palsy. *Arch. Phys. Therapy,* 23:332-336, June 1942.
PHELPS, W. M. AND JAMES, ROBERTIN: The prevention of postural deformities in children with cerebral palsy. *Arch. Phys. Med.,* 29: April 1948.
RUSK, HOWARD A.: Dynamic therapeutics in chronic disease. *New York State J. Med.,* 48:14:1597, July 15, 1948.
―――――――――――――:Rehabilitation of the Hemiplegic patient. *Internat. J. Neurol.,* 1:2:191-198, March 1960.
―――――――――――――: *Rehabilitation Medicine. A Textbook on Physical Medicine and Rehabilitation.* St. Louis, C. V. Mosby Co., 1958.
TEMPLE, FAY: The use of pathological and unlocking reflexes in the rehabilitation of spastics. *Am. J. Phys. Med.,* 33:No. 6, Dec. 1954, 347-352.
―――――――――――――: The neurophysical aspects of therapy in cerebral palsy: *Arch. Phys. Med.,* 29:6, June 1948.

Chapter 9

RESPIRATION

INDICATIONS

Proper breathing should always be maintained in all exercises in which any effort is expended and respiration thereby affected. In many instances, breathing exercises are indicated as a *part* of exercise programs; for certain pulmonary conditions, such as asthma, emphysema, and after chest surgery, such exercises form the core of the program.

Breathing exercises should be part of exercise therapy for poor posture, lesion of the central nervous system, such as poliomyelitis, certain types of cerebral palsy, and of a relaxation program.

As with other exercises, we are dealing with striated muscle and have to take into account its various physiological and pathological aspects, as pointed out in previous chapters. There is, however, one notable difference: the fact that the normal breathing process is subconscious, while it may be influenced by volition, it is only partly and to a limited extent amenable to commands.

It is possible, to accelerate breathing to a very fast pace, but at a certain point we shall have to stop; not because the muscles have become fatigued, but because saturation of the blood with oxygen forces us to stop. On the other hand, we can cease breathing, "hold our breath," by an act of will; but here again there is a certain moment when the blood, this time deprived of oxygen and overloaded with carbon dioxide, will by subcortical reflex force us to start breathing once more.

Breathing exercises may try first, to strengthen breathing muscles after they have been weakened or relax and stretch them if needed, and, second, that of teaching "breathing habits" different from those hitherto used by the patient and found inadequate.

Formative Influence on the Chest

The steadily repeated movements that form part of breathing may influence the formation of the chest and posture. Temporary or permanent elimination of one side of the thorax from breathing may produce deformities, especially during growing years. In these cases, asymmetry of the chest can be found, with one side smaller and lagging in excursion as compared to the other.

Normal breathing should be done by both chest and abdomen, that is, it should be mixed breathing, in about equal amounts. There should be approximately fifteen to twenty respirations (inhalations and expirations) in one minute when at rest. The muscles immediately concerned with breathing—intercostal muscles and diaphragm—are named respiratory muscles, and the muscles called upon to increase respiration in case of need —the scaleni, the pectoral muscles, the anterior serratus muscles and the abdominal muscles—are termed auxiliary respiratroy muscles.

One cannot directly influence intercostal muscles or the diaphragm, because they function as part of the breathing pattern and in normal respiration are used unconsciously in such a pattern. However, the auxiliary muscles (or at least some of them) act or volition and therefore respond to direct approach. Before breathing exercises are prescribed, a local appraisal of "breathing muscles" should be made. In case of chest disease, exercise prescription will have to take into account existing pathology.

Examination of the chest, preceding breathing exercises, should cover:

Shape of chest, chest excursion. The chest may be barrel-shaped, as in emphysema, and may show deep inspiration and poor expiration.

The chest may be long and "asthenic," flat, showing poor inspiration and poor expiration. It may move little, the main respiration being done by abdominal breathing. The patient may be a chest breather, doing main breathing with the chest.

Breathing should be observed in prone, sitting and standing positions. Fluoroscopic examination will give information about diaphragmatic breathing. The patient should inhale deeply and exhale deeply to expose deficiencies in either of these phases of respiration. It is sometimes necessary to watch respiration before and after physical activities. It may be measured by taking the circumference of the thorax at the apex of the sternum in middle and maximum positions of inspiration, and at maximum of expiration; these measurements are then compared with later results. Spirometric readings may be helpful and are an easy method of observing improvement of breathing.

In special weaknesses of the respiratory muscles the presence of contractures or muscle spasm must be noted, and may present the main problem, as in poliomyelitis, cerebral palsies or local chest pathology.

Following are a few special aspects of breathing exercises: In addition to those cases in which breathing may need separate attention, proper breathing should be observed when all special and general exercises are given. The most frequently made mistakes are tensing of the chest and auxiliary muscles and straining, particularly when the exercise performed requires a severe effort. Lack of complete expiration is the second most common fault. The therapist will therefore watch for relaxed breathing and for complete exhaling. These must be demonstrated to the patient and told to them one after the other because it is usually difficult for the patient to correct his bad habits.

The aims of breathing exercises are purposely simplified in the following categories:

TECHNIQUE

Breathing Muscles Proper
Chest, Intercostals, Diaphragm

Since, as already mentioned, these muscles do not normally respond directly to volitional impulses, they can be exercised only by performing the act of breathing in an intentionally modified form. When these muscles are not strong enough to perform unaided, the auxiliary muscles come into play. It should be part of training, however, gradually to eliminate substitution of this kind.

1. *Lack of muscle strength* as evidenced by *weak, incomplete inspiration*.
   A. Bilateral
      a. Supine. Inhale through the nose, if necessary with the assistance of auxiliary muscles, that is, holding on to the sides of a bed. Relax at expiration.
      b. Same as (a) above, sitting.
      c. Supine. Inhale trying to expand abdomen while inhaling (diaphragmatic breathing).
   B. Unilateral
      If one side of the thorax is lacking and requires increased inspiration, the patient should be placed on the opposite side, and Exercise A (a), as above, given with the patient lying on that side. Arm swing above the head may sometimes be added at inspiration, when the auxiliary muscles are used.
2. *Lack of elasticity* of the respiratory muscle proper may produce poor expiration. If this lack of elasticity is very marked, as in pronounced diaphragmatic spasm, inspiration may be considerably impaired also. If respiration is markedly impaired by acute painful spasm (as in poliomyelitis), the use of hot packs is indicated to relieve the spasm. Exercises should aim first at relaxation of the respiratory muscles, which may be obtained by:
   a. Shallow, easy and frequent breathing for a short period of time; rest for a while; return to previous shallow fast breathing.
   b. Regions of the chest and abdomen not otherwise used by the patient may be called upon to take over; concentrating on them by indirect relaxation may cause the others to relax. For instance, abdominal breathing if given to a normal chest breather may increase relaxation of breathing muscles by distracting the patient's attention.

When mainly expiration is impaired, breathing exercises should emphasize volitional expiration. Since expiration is normally done by inherent elasticity of the thorax rather than by muscle contraction, the stress on expiration requires the auxiliary muscles to contract and thus works for indirect relaxation of the respiratory muscles proper. Indirect relaxation can be produced by concentrating on breathing patterns hitherto not present in the patient's habits, on resistance, hard blowing out of air, hissing through the teeth, blowing up paper bags, etc.—all of which teach the patient to decrease the volume of thorax, an action not usually performed in normal breathing.

The following exercises have this aim:
- a. Lie on back, inhale through nose without special effort, exhale with hissing noise through teeth and prolong act of exhalation as far as possible.
- b. Same as (a) above, with emphasis on contraction of abdominal muscles.
- c. Same as (a) above, with arms above head at inhalation, crossed over chest and pressed down at exhalation. These exercises can be increased by performance in sitting and standing positions.

EXERCISES FOR AUXILIARY BREATHING MUSCLES

Scaleni, Pectorals, Anterior Serratus, Abdominals

Auxiliary breathing muscles may be constantly overworked if normal breathing is interfered with. They may then be very tensed and foreshortened and may require relaxation as well as active and passive stretching. For example:
1. Lie on back, abduct arms on inspiration as far as possible, adduct with expiration.
2. Abduct arms against resistance.
3. Elevate arms in supine position, with assistance and resistance.
4. Add gentle passive stretch to exercises 1, 2, 3.

Breathing Exercises as Part of Other Exercise Programs
Posture Exercises

Breathing exercises in connection with posture training should correct poor breathing habits such as excessive and exaggerated chest breathing, shallow breathing, lack of even respiration when moving or doing the exercises, and excessive abdominal breathing. The exercises are part of the posture program as a whole. Unilateral breathing, especially unilateral chest breathing, should be given to most scoliosis cases.

Exercises

(A) *Double Breathing:* Patient lying on back, hands locked behind head, knees flexed: breathe in through nose raising ribs (relaxed shoulders). Breathe out through mouth, lowering ribs as far as possible, making a hissing sound.

(A) *Breathing with Lateral Arm Swing:* Patient lying on back, arms at side of body, knees flexed. Swing arms over head and sideways, breathing in through nose, stretch, breathe out through mouth, hissing, swinging arms down. Relax.

(A) *Breathing with Forward Arm Swing:* Same as above, but swinging arms forward and overhead.

(A) *Prone Breathing:* Patient lying prone, head resting on folded arms. Breathe in through nose, breathe out through mouth with hissing sound, physical therapist helping patient to exhale and to lower ribs. Relax.

(A) *One-sided Breathing in Lateral Position:* Patient lying on right or left side over flat hard pillow placed under ribs. Right or left arm with bent elbow over head. Breathe in through nose, breathe out through mouth with hissing sound. Relax (Fig. 86).

(A) *Abdominal Breathing:* Patient on back, arms at sides, knees flexed. Breathe in and out, raising and lowering abdomen, with or without resisting weight on abdomen.

(A) *Standing Breathing:* Patient standing, leans forward, arms dangling. Stretch arms overhead, rising to erect position on toes, breathing in. Drop forward, breathing out through mouth making a hissing sound. Relax. Repeat (Fig. 87).

(B) *Chest and Abdominal Breathing:* Position as in *Abdominal Breathing:* Breathe in through nose, expanding abdomen, then chest. Breathe out through mouth making a hissing sound, lowering abdomen, then chest.

Poliomyelitis

In the acute stage of poliomyelitis, there may be spasm of the respiratory muscles, and this will require the use of hot packs. If respiratory muscle power is impaired, breathing exercises

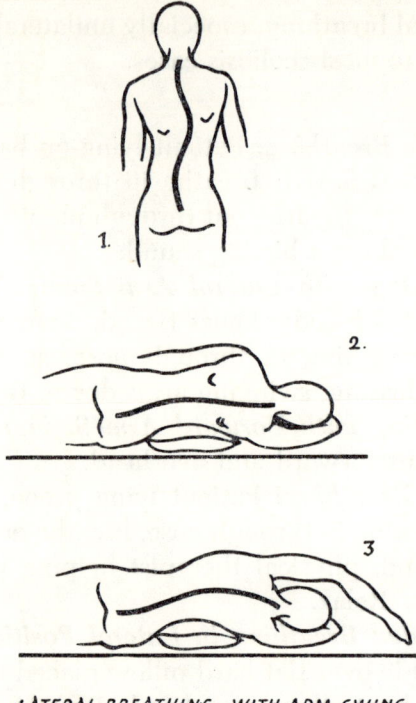

LATERAL BREATHING WITH ARM SWING

Fig. 86

should start as soon as possible, keeping in mind the patient's general condition. These should be as follows:
1. Supine. Inhale through nose, exhale while relaxing.
2. Supine. Inhale, trying to expand abdomen while inhaling, exhale while relaxing.
3. Supine. Inhale through nose, exhale through teeth with hissing sound as long as possible.
4. Supine. Place palms on chest. Inhale. Exhale, while pressing palms on chest to make it possible to exhale as much as possible. Stress should be placed on even inspiration. Relaxation should be stressed in most cases, even if no muscle spasm has been present, because respiratory muscles worked at maximum and not at optimum may frequently tend to tighten.

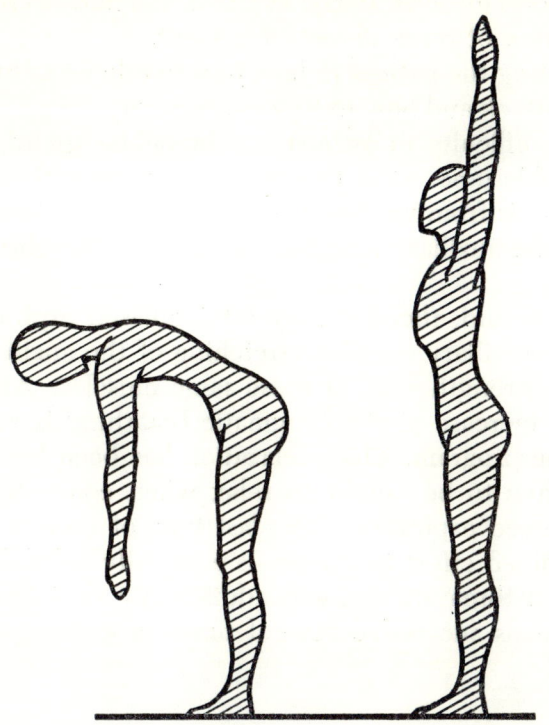

STANDING BREATHING WITH ARM SWING

Fig. 87

Cerebral Palsy

Breathing exercises may be necessary in all types of cerebral palsies as a preliminary for speech training or to produce general relaxation. In athetosis the teaching of even, relaxed expiration is of special importance. In general relaxation for athetoids, volitional breathing is a useful technique to bring about relaxation by distracting attention from other volitional acts.

Special Pulmonary Conditions
Asthma

Some of the aims of breathing exercises for asthma are:
1. *Prevention* of the accompanying postural defects, such as

shortened pectoral muscles, dorsal kyphosis and narrowed chest.

2. *Correction* of these defects if present.

3. Instructing the patient in how best to relieve asthma, how to prevent an attack and how to lessen its severity.

The main difficulty in asthma is a bronchial spasm, making expiration troublesome. It is this obstacle to expiration, the inability to expel air from the lungs, that produces the tensing and shortening of the auxiliary muscles and narrows the chest excursion.

Exercises should, therefore, try for increased expiration, relaxation of the auxiliary muscles, stretching of the auxiliary muscles as well as strengthening of these same muscles. Abdominal breathing and increase of diaphragmatic breathing is an important part of the program. Once relaxation has been learned, the patient will have to be taught to relax when concentrating on increasingly forced expiration. The last type of exercise—relaxation plus combined effort to exhale—is especially helpful in stopping incipient asthma attacks, and additionally so if the patient has by this means succeeded several times in getting some immediate relief.

Exercises

1. Supine. Arms at sides. Knees flexed. Breathe in and out, raising and lowering abdomen (Fig. 88).

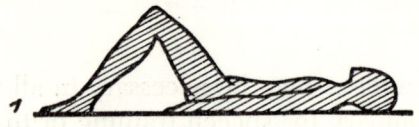
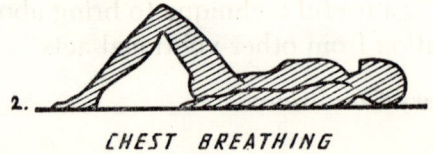

CHEST BREATHING

Fig. 88

2. Supine. Position as in (1). Breathe in through nose, expanding abdomen first, then chest. Breathe out through teeth, making a hissing sound, lowering abdomen first, then chest.
3. Standing. Patient leans forward, arms dangling. Stretch arms overhead, rising to erect position on toes—inhale. Drop forward, exhaling through teeth making hissing sound.

In Emphysema

In Emphysema the volume of the lungs is unduly enlarged, the thorax "blown up," and expiration markedly reduced. Measurement of medium inspiration may reveal a very large chest with relatively small excursions, showing that both inspiration and expiration have suffered. Appropriate exercises are:
1. Supine. Inhale through nose, exhale while relaxing, being conscious of exhaling.
2. Supine. Inhale through nose, exhale with hissing noise through teeth.
3. Supine. Inhale through nose, exhale while trying to pull abdomen up and in. Put palm on abdomen for contrast.
4. Prone. Head resting on crossed arms. Inhale through nose, exhale through teeth with hissing noise, therapist helping patient to exhale by pressing on lower ribs.

The tendency will be to increase expiration, and secondarily, to improve respiration. Relaxation of the auxiliary muscles will quite often be necessary, and relaxed breathing, as well as abdominal breathing, may need to be trained.

After Operation

After surgery, breathing is a subject for special attention. It is worthwhile to teach proper breathing, coughing and expectorating pre-operatively, and to train the patient to do chest breathing if abdominal surgery is planned, making abdominal breathing painful.

In chest surgery, breathing exercises are particularly important. If possible, breathing should be taught and exercised pre-operatively, in both supine and sitting positions. Auxiliary breathing should be taught; if the operation may eliminate one side of the chest for a certain period, unilateral breathing of the opposite side should be stressed and specially trained. Abdominal breathing ought also to be taught. Coughing and expectorating should be trained whenever possible.

Post-operatively, the program depends largely on the surgery performed and the particular requirements of the case. As soon as possible, shallow breathing and then deeper chest and abdominal breathing should be done several times a day for short periods. There should be active and passive abduction and elevation of the arms to prevent contractions of the shoulder girdle muscles. General convalescent exercises are to be added as soon as possible.

1. Supine. Inhale through nose, exhale while relaxing.
2. Supine. Inhale through nose, trying to expand abdomen, exhale while relaxing.
3. Supine. Arms at sides, knees flexed. Inhale and exhale while raising and lowering abdomen.
4. Supine. Same position as in 3. Inhale through nose, expanding abdomen first, then chest. Exhale through teeth, making hissing noise, lowering first abdomen, then chest.
5. Supine. Inhale while arms are raised over head. Exhale while crossing them on chest.
6. Supine. Inhale while abducting arms. Exhale while adducting. Can be performed active, with assistance, with resistance, with resistance given to abductors of arms.

RECOMMENDED READING

BAKER, FRANCES: Exercise in the treatment of asthma. *Arch. Phys. Med.,* XXXII: No. 1, Jan. 1951.

BARRACH, ALVIN L.: Breathing exercises in pulmonary emphysema and allied chronic respiratory disease. *Arch. Phys. Med. & Rehab.,* 36: No. 6, p. 379, June, 1955.

SCHMITT, JOHANNES L.: *Atemheilkunst.* Berlin, H. J. Muller Verlag, 1956.

SCHUTZ, KARL: Exercise in therapy of bronchial asthma. *Mod. Med.,* p. 102, June 15, 1955.

PART 3
GENERAL EXERCISES

PART 3
GENERAL EXERCISES

Chapter 10

GENERAL EXERCISES
INDICATIONS, DOSAGE

EXERCISES FOR localized difficulties must be *directed* to as small areas of the body as possible in order to utilize all exercise time toward the desired end. *Local* exercises, therefore, have little effect on the whole body. With *general* exercises, the opposite is true; for the aim is to influence the *whole* organism: circulation, breathing, general muscle strength, relaxation, metabolism and digestion. The general effect of exercises has been studied and is well known. However, it is still not widely enough used for therapeutic purposes. There are still too many occasions of the transition from prolonged bed-rest to walking consisting of only a few days of sitting in a wheelchair. Exercises to keep patients in good physical condition during prolonged bed-rest are equally neglected. Pre- and post-operative exercises before and after childbirth, exercises for cardiacs, exercises after surgery, etc., have yet to be accepted as an integral part of the treatment program.

The general exercises for the various conditions mentioned in the following pages are not specific, and differ in local aims from exercises already described. A minor problem of local character, such as special weakness of legs, tightness of certain muscle groups produced by long bed rest, poor breathing, etc. may be present, but such a local problem may be only a part of the larger one of improving the general condition of the patient. The local problem should continue to be treated according to the principles and suggestions presented in earlier chapters.

Sometimes the local problem is more serious; it may even constitute the main problem of the case. Rheumatoid arthritis, disabilities produced by burns with ensuing scars, post-operative scars, contractures after prolonged immobilization, such as adduction contraction of humerus after mastectomy or after long bedrest in coronary disease, may cause local problems of muscle function and joint motion. Such cases require, treatment of the cause, and as soon as possible, local treatment as well as general convalescent exercise.

The principles of local treatment have been discussed in section on the musculo-skeletal system. Treatment and needs of the basic pathology should determine any necessary modifications.

Since the exercises given for this group of cases are on the whole of a general character, the prescription differs accordingly. Dosage is of as much interest as before—that is, the time and intensity of the exercises—but the dosage should consist of the total of *all* exercises required. It is necessary to repeat that we are not interested in *directing* our efforts towards *one particular* region of the body: on the contrary, the exercises should be distributed with a view towards a complete workout for the body. For instance, all joints should go through the full range of motion; all muscles should contract and relax and cover the full range of activity. Grade the exercises according to the needs and capacities of the individual patient. In cases of weak patients in poor condition, provide for scattered dosage of very low grade exercises, to be gradually increased to short periods of more intense activity. A general workout rather than any specialized movement should always be kept in mind.

General fatigue and strain on circulation need to be watched for, rather than *local* fatigue.

Masters' test offers a method of determining cardio-vascular exercise tolerance; it is carried out as follows: The patient is made to take two steps up and two steps down, each step of nine inches, after the patient has rested and his pulse and blood pressure have become stable. The patient is then made to walk up and down these steps for 90 seconds. The speed of his performance has been established depending on age, sex and wight, and these figures have been arranged on an exercise tolerance table by Masters. Pulse rate and blood pressure should return to normal in 2 minutes. This test can, of course, not be applied to bedridden patients or to those with very low exercise tolerance.

An *example follows of a general exercise program for a pa-*

tient with bed rest; it is an example only—to be modified according to the individual case:

Exercise periods—five minutes to 15 minutes, 1-3 times a day.
1. Flexion and extension of all joints, done in alternate extremities. For example: flexion and extension of toes of left foot, flexion and extension of toes of fingers of left hand, flexion and extension of fingers of right hand. Repeat for wrist, elbow and shoulder, ankles, knees and hips.
2. Add breathing exercises—deep inspiration and complete expiration, (a) chest, (b) abdominal.
3. Add abduction of both arms at inspiration and crossing of both arms over chest at expiration.
4. Tensing of abdominal muscles.
5. Turning over in bed.
6. Flexion of all joints against gravity by raising extremity off the bed.
7. As above, plus weight of one or two pounds for each extremity.
8. Elevation of body, aided at first by bar. Dispense with bar when no longer necessary.

Convalescent Exercises

Regular exercise periods for a patient in bed should be started as soon as possible and should attempt to keep the patient and the musculature and joints in the best general condition possible. The exercise aim is to maintain and increase muscle strength and muscle elasticity, promote general and local circulation and adequate ventilation of the lungs.

Contractures should always be avoided in patients undergoing bed rest by bringing the joints through the full range, passively if necessary, at least once a day and by positioning the extremities at an advantageous angle. It is important to keep the ankles in a 90° flexed position. The feet should not be subject to the constant pressure of a heavy blanket. Likewise it is important to prevent flexion contracture in joints, including the hip joint. *Frequent turning and maintaining prone position for longer periods at a time should be encouraged. The practice of "tucking in" patients limits the ability to move and should be abandoned.*

The exercises outlined above usually achieve this purpose; most of the modes of procedure indicated thus far should be observed. Exercises must be given within fatique limits, and below pain limits if there is pain, and in appropriate dosage. The program should be curtailed and scattered in more severe cases, and concentrated and increased in less severe ones.

Exercise must always be performed slowly through the full range of motion, with a rest period for relaxation after the motion has been completed. If these exercises are intensified as a preliminary to sitting up and walking, the convalescent period in bed can be considerably shortened. If there is particular weakness in the legs, strengthening of the lower extremities should be stressed. Should crutch walking be necessary, special strengthening of the upper extremities, especially the triceps, should be prescribed.

Special requirements for local and general exercise differ according to the case:

Surgery: After abdominal operation, breathing exercises and, as soon as possible, abdominal breathing should be given attention. Leg and foot exercises begun at the earliest possible moment can go a long way toward preventing complications from thromboses of the veins of the legs.*

After removal of the breast for cancer, limitation of shoulder motion and swelling of the upper extremity can be prevented or minimized if exercises to preserve and increase abduction of the shoulder and exercises to preserve strength and range of the elbow and hand are initiated as soon as surgically permissible. These should begin with scattered dosage.

After plastic operations, local problems of limitation of joint motion and of atrophy from inactivity require localized as well as general exercise.

Tendon plastics and tendon sutures need mobilization, as soon as possible.

In minor surgery, especially involving the extremities, early

---

*Burger exercises are used to improve the circulation of the lower extremities. The legs are elevated to 45° for 2 minutes, lowered over the edge of the bed for 3 minutes, during which time ankle flexion, extension, supination, pronation, toe spreading and closing is performed, and finally the legs are rested in a horizontal position for 5 minutes.

active and passive motion is called for, and it should never be overlooked after surgery to hand and fingers.

Pulmonary operations require breathing exercises as well as general ones. In chest surgery, good pre-operative preparation is important.

The *pre-operative* preparation of the patient for the post-operative position is helpful. This procedure has been described in detail under othopedic conditions, and holds good, of course, for operations on the trunk as well as those on the extremities. When parts of the body are to be permanently or temporarily out of use after an operation, compensation by other parts is worth attempting. Strengthening the abdominal walls can help prevent post-operative constipation.

In *obstetrics*, general exercises to preserve a good physical condition before delivery have been found of advantage by many obstetricians. The stress is laid on strengthening abdominal muscles and pelvic muscles, but equally there should be training for general strength and elasticity. Stretching of adductors of thigh and posture training are included. Foot and leg exercises may prepare for the expected increase in weight. Relaxation and breathing exercises are part of the "natural childbirth" programs.

A sizeable number of low back complaints in women date from pregnancy, and in many cases these complaints are accompanied by weak abdominal muscles and, at times, exaggerated lumbar lordosis (increased pelvic tilt). Abdominal strengthening and pelvic straightening exercises should always be included in pre- and post-natal routine and will help to prevent back pain.

In geriatrics well balanced exercises are an essential part of the management.

Prolonged bed rest in *cardiac cases* should be combined with an adequate bed exercise program. Exercises such as those outlined on page 233 may be used on a scattered basis as soon as they can be done without the patient's showing fatigue, increased pulse rate or breathing difficulties. When starting exercises for a bedridden patient, the transition from lying to sitting and finally to standing is of significance. This is especially true for cardiac patients. It is not enough to grade the exercises for these cases according to effort. It is necessary to select the exercises for lying position with low energy cost at the beginning, and only later and gradually to progress to those for upright position. They should be increased little by little and worked up very slowly until the day when the patient may sit up. The usual method of having a patient sit up and dangle his feet over the edge of the bed, after a prolonged period in bed, then of allowing him up in a chair for an increasing period during the day and then of starting ambulation, is an exceedingly violent and fast program for the cardiac patient compared with the prolonged and gradually developing exercise program in lying position that can slowly prepare for such efforts.

Once the cardiac patient is up and around, an exercise program that increases by very slow degrees can improve circulation and general resistance to a point where the patient may be able to extend activities considerably.

In *obesity*, exercises are often prescribed as an adjunct to diet. Circulation and respiration need to be watched with particular care. It is difficult to give strenuous, calorie-consuming exercises to a fat person who is at the same time under reducing medication, without there being a marked effect on the general circulation. The speed of the exercises may have to be accelerated beyond that normally prescribed, because speed of performance increases calory requirement; walking only burns 110 calories per hour, while light exercise requires 535. In case dehydration of the patient by medication is sought as a means of weight reduction, muscle cramps may occur if further dehydration is produced by sweating during exercise. Excessive dehydration of this kind must be watched for when exercises are given for weight reduction.

Teaching abdominal contraction has been found worthwhile in cases of *constipation*. Abdominal exercises for constipation should, however, be compined with general exercises.

EXERCISES FOR NERVOUS TENSION

Another type of general exercise is that for "nervous tension." Since the mind's only outlet is the striated muscle, whatever disturbs a person is reflected in muscle action. If irritations, be they

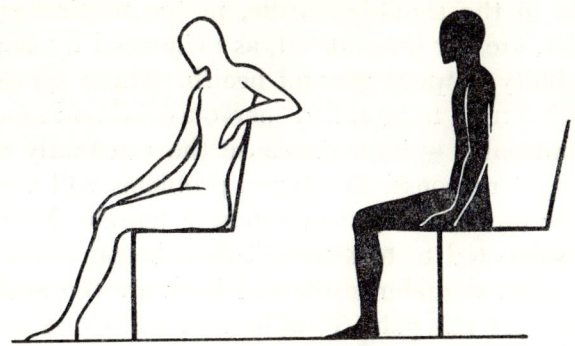

MUSCLES ARE THE ONLY MEANS
TO EXPRESS MIND —
THEY REFLECT "MENTAL TENSENESS
OR RELAXATION."

Fig. 89

emotional or extrinsic, recur daily and establish similar patterns of response, it can be readily understood that an habitual pattern of muscular reaction is formed.

This pattern is, to a large degree, influenced by daily activities. The regional distribution of muscle tenseness will depend on occupation, educational background and opportunity to give motor outlet to emotional strain (Fig. 89). Since all these factors are geared to inhibit motor responses, and since physical training usually teaches how to contract but not how to release contraction, it is clear why all these factors lead to local or generalized isometric muscle contraction—tenseness without the relief of resulting action. This fact has been recognized only within the past decades, and exercises for progressive relaxation have only recently been introduced (Jacobson: *Progressive Relaxation*).

Relaxation should be included in all exercise curricula, especially for city-dwellers or people engaged in work requiring a high degree of self-restraint, tension and ability to stand up to mental pressure. Every growing individual should be taught that muscle action consists not only of contraction but also of giving up contraction, i.e., relaxing. Once the state of tension has reached the borderline of physiology, it can become either more localized, for example in the shoulder girdle, in the respiratory muscles, neck muscles, etc., or generalized, as evidenced by sleeplessness, hyper-irritability or poor general health. These symptoms may add up to what used to be called "nervousness" and more recently "tension syndrome" — its main cause the constantly suppressed fight and flight response. Emotional problems will contribute to these outside forces and produce muscle tension. Muscle groups frequently subjected to tension will then become stiff and painful. Head, neck, shoulder girdle and back are the most frequent "target areas" for this pain. Tension pain will cause anxiety, and anxiety will cause tension thus closing the vicious cycle. It has been shown that by teaching a person how to relax, this complex can be immensely relieved, and that muscular relaxation may in addition help to relieve muscular tension.

General progressive relaxation is accomplished by placing the patient in a comfortable recumbent position, and first teaching him the difference between contraction and relaxation by letting him contract some of his muscles (e.g. the biceps) and then teaching how to give up this contraction (direct relaxation).

Indirect relaxation can also be used from the start by having the patient concentrate on his breathing and by teaching proper respiration, thereby distracting attention from other parts of his body and improving his state of relaxation. From then on, relaxation should, as described before, be trained with passive movement, active movement and active movement against gravity, with the patient in less comfortable lying positions and finally sitting and standing.

Regional relaxation may be required for individuals whose tenseness is concentrated in special areas, and habit forming relaxation movements should be prescribed, such as relaxation of the shoulders at intervals during work, relaxation in breathing, relaxing of the neck muscles, etc.

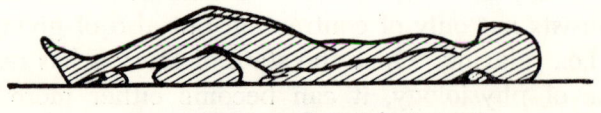

POSITION FOR RELAXATION

Fig. 90

A good heavy workout requiring effort and concentration is the best relaxing exercise. However, patients who are very tense may be unable to perform strenuous physical exercise without increasing tension in target areas and thereby producing pain. A general workout should, therefore, be preceded by relaxation, and a gradual warm-up and should end with cool off exercises and another period of breathing exercises.

Preventive Exercises

Our over-mechanized way of life deprives us of the minimum amount of exercise necessary for healthful living. There is increasing evidence that under-exercise is an important factor in ethiology of disease, ranging from coronary disease to back pain. Much has been done in other countries, such as Germany, Austria and Russia to prevent under exercise disease (Hypokinetic Disease).

Still healthy people showing the first signs of being overworked, overtensed, over fed and underexercised may go to treatment centers where they have opportunity to rest their minds and recondition their bodies under systematic exercise regimens. Nationwide fitness programs throughout the life of the individual are effective in these countries and have preventive value.

Physicians and therapists interested in therapeutic exercises will find it rewarding to extend their study and practice to normal gymnastics and exercises.

RECOMMENDED READING

ALTSCHULE, MARK D.: *Bodily Physiology in Mental and Emotional Disorders*. New York, Grune & Stratton, 1953.
BECKMANN, P.: Die Bewegungsbehandlung bei Inneren Krankheiten. Die Therapie-Wohe, May, 1960.
———————:Die Hypokinetschen Erkrankungen und die Muskeluntersuchung. Hyprocrates, 31, Jahrgang, Heft 10, 31, May, 1960.
———————: Fruehbehandlung von Herz- und Kreislaufschaeden. Aerztliche Praxis, XII. Jahrgang, No. 40, pp. 1935, 1959-1963, 1, Oct. 1960.
CANNON, WALTER B.: The mechanism of emotional disturbance of bodily functions. *New England J. Med.*, pp. 877-884, 1928.
CLARK, H. HARRISON: *Development of the Sub-Strength Individual*. Fred Medart Products, Inc., St. Louis, 1951.
GORDON, EDWARD E.: Energy costs in prescription of activity. *Mod. Med.*, 25: No. 24, 83-91, 1957.

———————————: Energy cost of activities in health and disease. *AMA Arch. Int. Med.*, *101*:702-713, April, 1958.

HAUGEN, G. B., DIXON, H. H. AND DICKEL, H. A.: A Therapy for Anxiety Tension Reaction. New York, The Macmillan Co.

HAWKINS, MARY O'NEILL: Exercise and emotional stability. *Child Study*, 33: No. 2, pp. 7-10, Spring, 1956.

HEADY, J. A., MORRIS, J. N., LLOYD, F. J. AND RAFFLE, P. A. B.: Sickness absence before the first clinical episode of coronary heart disease. *Brit. J. Indust. Med.*, *11*:20, 1954.

HOLMSTROEM, A.: *Swedish Gymnastics Today*. Stockholm, Sohlmans Foerlag, 1949.

JACOBSON, EDMUND: *Progressive Relaxation*. Chicago, Univ. of Chicago Press, 1938.

KIPHUTH, ROBERT J. H.: *How To Be Fit*. New Haven, Yale Univ. Press, 1960.

KLUMPP, THEODORE G.: Heart Attacks Not Due to Physical Exertion. Winthrop Lab., 1450 Broadway, NYC, Nov. 27, 1957.

KRAUS, HANS AND RAAB, W.: *Hypokinetic Disease: Diseases Produced by Lack of Exercise*. Springfield, Thomas, 1961.

KRAUS, HANS AND HIRSCHLAND, RUTH P.: Minimum muscular fitness tests in school children. *Res. Quart.*, *25*:2, pp. 178- 188, May 1954.

LANE, W. KENNETH: Role of pediatrician in physical fitness of youth. *J. A. M. A.*, Jan. 1959, *169*:221-227, Jan. 1959.

MAYER, JEAN: Exercise does keep the weight down. *Atlantic Monthly*, 1955.

MORRIS, J. N. AND HEADY, T. H., ET AL.: Coronary Heart Disease by Under-Exercise. *Lancet*, 1953.

RAAB, W.: Loafer's heart (Das Faulenzerherz). *AMA Arch. Int. Med.*, *101*:194-198, Feb. 1958. *Wiener Klin. Wochenschrift.*, No. 38/39, pp. 709-711, 1958.

———————————: Hazards of a Loafers Civilization. Are We Loafing Our Hearts to Death?

RIVOIRE, M. R., RIVOIRE, J. AND POUJOL, M. J.: La fatigue: syndrome d' insuffisance surrenale fonctionelle. *Press Med.*, *61*:1431, Nov. 4, 1953.

SELYE, HANS: *The Story of the Adaptation Syndrome*. Montreal, Canada, Med. Publishers, 1952.

TWOMBLY, G. C.: Pre- and post-partum exercise techniques, indications, benefits. *Arch. Phys. Med. & Rehab.*, p. 632, Dec. 1960.

WHITE, PAUL D.: The Ways of Life and Heart Disease. *Harvard Med. Alumni Bull.*, Oct. 1956.

INDEX

A

Abdominal breathing, 223
Abdominal exercises, 110-112
Abdominal muscles, 219, 222
   strength of, 104-106
   strengthening exercises for, 127-128
Accomplishment
   exercises, 201
   tests, 36-37, 38, 201
     of balance, 36
Accordion exercise, 116
Acromioclavicular dislocation, 142
Active-assistive exercise, 41
Adhesions
   capsular, 34
   fibrous, 160, 167
   pericapsular, 34
Aeroplane exercise, 114
Alarm reaction, 22
Anesthetics, surface, 62-67, 96
   in ankle sprains, 171
   in back pain, 132
   in neck injuries, 135
   in upper extremity pain, 138
Ankle
   dorsiflexion of, 16, 206
   exercise, 170-173
   fractures of, 170
   sprain of, 170-173
Apparatus for exercise, 53-54
Arches
   relaxation of, 173
   support of, 175
Arm
   raising exercise, 119, 129
   rotation exercise, 113
   spread exercise, 113
   stretch, sitting, 119
Arthritis
   exercise in, 95, 125
   of hipjoint, 155-156
   of knee joint, 166-168
   of wrist, 150
Arthroplasty of hip, exercise after, 154
Assistive exercises, 41
   for strength-building, 45-46
Asthma, 225-227
Ataxia, 210-211
   adult, 216
   coordination exercises in, 51
   in tabes dorsalis, 200
Athetosis, 211-212
   relaxation in, 50
Athletic activities, injury from, 83-86
Atrophy, 12, 16
Attitude of patient, 86-87, 94
Auxiliary respiratory muscles, 219, 222-224
Axillary nerve injury, 183-184

B

Back
   kneeling back pull, 113
   mobility and rotation, exercises for, 114-115
   pain, 124-135
     acute, 132-135
     causes of, 79-81, 124
     exercises for, 99
     palpation in, 126
     strengthening exercises, 127-129
     stretching exercises, 129-132
     tests in, 125-126
   strength of muscles, 106
Balance accomplishments, 36, 51
Ball games, injuries in, 85, 86
Baseball, injuries in, 85
Basketball, injury from, 86
Baths, hot, 62, 193
Bed exercises, 233, 235

Bell's palsy, 185
Bend over exercise, standing, 115
Braces
  in muscle dystrophies, 190
  in paraplegia, 198
  in sciatic nerve lesions, 186, 187
  in spastic paralysis, 212
Brachial plexus injuries, 188
Brassieres, pain from, 79
Breathing
  adbominal, 223
  auxiliary muscles in, 219, 222-224
  exercises, 109-110, 218-228
    in asthma, 225-227
    in cerebral palsy, 225
    in emphysema, 227
    in poliomyelitis, 195, 223-224
    postoperative, 227-228, 234
    posture exercises with, 222-223
  formative influence on chest, 219-220
  observation of, 107
Bridge
  abdominal, 111
  body, 114
Bursitis of shoulder
  acute, 143-145
  chronic, 145

C

Calcium deposits, 143
Calf muscles, strained, 169
Callus formation, 91, 184
Camphor liniment, after ethyl chloride spray, 63
Cardiac disease, exercise in, 235
Catback exercise, 129
Cerebral palsies, 201-212
  breathing exercises in, 225
  relaxation in, 51
Cervical spine, 135-137
Chairs, relaxation, 204, 212
Chest
  examination of, 219
  expansion of, 101, 107
Children
  brachial plexus injuries, 188
  cerebral palsies, 201-212

  exercises for, 25, 44, 47 (*see also* Conditioning exercise)
  foot conditions, chronic, 173-174
  poliomyelitis, 191-197
  postural dificiencies, 83
  pseudo-hypertrophy of muscle, 189-190
  torticollis, congenital, 136-137
Clavicle, fracture of, 138-140
Clothing habits, effects of, 77-81
Collars, pain from, 79
Colles fracture, 149
Conditioned reflexes, 25
Conditioning exercises, 25-26, 44, 205
  for relaxation, 50-51
  for strength-building, 47
Confusion movements, 16, 206
Constipation, exercises in, 236
Contraction, 5, 7
  concentric, 11
  de-contraction, 18
  eccentric, 9
  isometric, 8
Contracture, 20, 22, 56
  grading of, 35
  prevention of, 233
  stretching in, 23-24
  in tension states, 59
Convalescent exercises, 233-236
Co-ordination, 6, 7, 24-27
  after fractures, 93
  development of, 26-27
  exercises for, 51-53, 200-201
  measurement of, 36-38
  pathology of, 26
  physiology of, 24-26
Crutch paralysis, 184
Crutch walking, 137
Curare, use of, 193

D

Deconcentration, 50
Decontraction, 18
De Lorme method, 46, 165
Deltoid muscle paralysis, 183
Diaphragm, 219, 220
  in poliomyelitis, 195
Diplegia, 204

Dislocation
    acromioclavicular, 142
    elbow joint, 147
    hip, congenital, 156-157
    shoulder joint, 142-143
Doorknob turning exercise, 113, 119
Dystrophies, muscle, 189-190

E

Elasticity, 5, 7, 18-24
    development of, 22-23
    exercises for, 48-51
    of gluteal muscles, 104, 108
    of hamstrings, 104, 108
    measurement of, 33-36
    pathology of, 20-24
    of pectoral muscles, 103, 108
    physiology of, 18-20
    relative, 38
    of respiratory muscle, lack of, 221
Elbow
    chronic injury to, 147-148
    dislocations of, 147
    tennis elbow, 85, 147
Emphysema, 227
Eudurance, 9, 33
    development of, 16
    diminished, 13
Erector spinae muscles, elasticity of, 104, 108
Ethyl chloride spray, 62-64 (see also Anesthetics, surface)
Exercise
    apparatus for, 53-54
    conditioning, 25-26, 44, 47, 50-51, 205
    general, 231-240
    group work, 53, 95
    for muscle strength, 13-18, 45-47 (see also Strength, exercises for)
    passive, 24, 40, 41
    period for, building of, 44-45
    for posture, 109, 222
    prescription for, 69-76, 77-87
    preventive, 239
    teaching of, 40-44
    techniques of, 40-54

tolerance test, 232
unilateral, 117-123
(see also specific exercises)
Expiration, impairment of, 221
Extension and flexion exercise, 110
Extremities
    lower, 152-176, 186
    upper, 137-152
Eye muscles, 195

F

Face muscles, 185, 195
Facial nerve paralysis, 185
Fatigue
    effects of, 32, 35
    limits of, 15
Fatigue-Training Graph, 13-15, 20
Femur fracture
    distal end, 161
    neck, 153-155
    shaft, 159-161
Fibrositis, 58, 98
    and neck pain, 136
    palpating for, 126
    and shoulder pain, 145
Fibula, fractured, 168-169
Fingers, fractured, 151
Flexion
    back, exercise for, 114
    exercises, 116
Flexion and extension
    exercise, 110
    of hip and knee, 131
Floor touch exercise, 131
Foot
    chronic conditions, 173-176
    exercises, 122
    fractures of, 173
Football, injury from, 86
Forearm, fracture of, 148-149
Fracture
    of ankle, 170
    of clavicle, 138-140
    Colles, 149
    of elbow joint, 146-147
    of femur
        distal end, 161
        neck, 153-155

shaft, 159-161
  of fibula, 168-169
  of fingers, 151
  of foot, 173
  of forearm, 148-149
  of humerus
    distal end, 146
    head, 140-142
    shaft, 146
  of metacarpals, 151
  of metatarsals, 173
  of patella, 161-162
  of radius, distal end, 149
  of spine, 99, 125, 133-135
  of tibia
    condyles, 168
    shaft, 168
  treatment of, 92-96
Frostbite, from ethyl chloride spray, 63
Functions of muscles, 5-8

G

Gastrocnemius
  strain of, 169
  stretch of, 110
General exercises, 231-240
Girdles, tight, 78
Gluteal muscles, elasticity of, 104, 108
Golf, injury from, 85
Goniometer, use of, 33
Gravity
  exercise against, 46
  relaxation against, 50
Group treatment, 53, 95

H

Habit-forming exercises, 52-53
Hamstring muscles
  acute injuries to, 157-159
  elasticity of, 104, 108
  stretch exercises, 115-116, 129-132
Heart disease, exercise in, 235
Heat, in pain, 61-62, 98
Heel slide exercise, 128
Hemiplegia, 204, 213
  spastic, 214-216
Hip
  arthritis of, 155-156
  dislocations, congenital, 156-157
  extension exercise, 122
  flexors, strengthening exercises for, 128
  injuries of, 153-159
  muscle injuries
    acute, 157-159
    chronic, 159
Histamine iontophoresis, 66
Holding power, 8, 33
  development of, 18
  measurements of, 104, 108
Humerus fracture
  distal end, 146
  head, 140-142
  shaft, 146
Hyper-tenseness, 22

I

Iliacus-psoas strength building, 121-122
Ilium, level of anterior-superior spines of, 101, 107
Incoordination, 26
Inspiration, impairment of, 221
Intercostal muscles, 219, 220
  in poliomyelitis, 195
Involuntary movement, 26-27
  gauging of, 37
Iontophoresis
  histamine, 66
  novocaine, 64, 143

J

Javelin throwing, injury from, 85
Jelling pain, in back, 124, 133
Joints, range of, 33

K

Knee
  arthritis of, 166
  chronic conditions of, 166-168
  injuries of, 161-168
  intra-articular injuries of, 162
  sprain of, 163-166

Knee kiss exercises, 111, 112, 128
Kneeling back pull exercise, 113
Kraus-Weber tests for muscular fitness, 125-126
Kyphosis, dorsal, 102, 108

L

Landmarks, measurement of, 38
Leg
    circle exercise, 112
    hold exercise, 112
    kick over head, 115
    length of, 102, 107
    paralysis of, 198
    raising exercise, 128
    swing over toward hand, 115
Look up-look back exercise, 119
Lordosis, lumbar, 102, 108
Lower extremities, 152-176
    peripheral nerve lesions, 186-188

M

Masters test, 232
Mattresses, types of, 79
Measurements, 29-39
    accomplishment tests, 36-37, 38
    of coordination, 36-38
    of elasticity, 33-36, 38
    functional, 103-104, 108
    of holding power, 104-106, 108
    of landmarks, 38
    motor-chain, 29-30
    recording of, 38-39
    regional function tests, 38
    requirements for tests, 30-31
    of strength, 31-33, 38, 104, 108
    structural, 101-103, 107
Medial nerve paralysis, 185
Metacarpal bones, fractured, 151
Metatarsal bones, fractured, 173
Monoplegia, 204
Morton toe, 175
Motor-chain
    measurements, 29-30
    pain in, 66
Motor retardations, 212-213
Movements, 25

confusion, 16, 206
involuntary, 26-27, 37
Muscle
    atrophy, 12, 16
    chart, 181-182
    dystrophies, 189-190
    function, 5-8
    pseudo-hypertrophy, 12, 189
    strength (*see* Strength, of muscles)
    testing of, 29-39
Musculo-skeletal apparatus, 91-178
    back pain, 124-135
    lower extremities, 152-176
    neck, 135-137
    posture, 100-123
    upper extremity, 137-152

N

Neck, 135-137
    acute conditions, 135
    chronic conditions, 136
    exercises for, 116-117
    torticollis, congenital, 136-137
Nerves, peripheral, 183-188
Nervous system, 179-217
    lower motor neuron lesions, 179, 181-201
    upper motor neuron lesions, 180, 201-216
Novocaine
    iontophoresis, 64
        in shoulder pain, 143
        in triggerpoints, 57

O

Obesity, exercisese in, 236
Obstetrics, exercises in, 235
Occupational hazards, 81-82
One-sided breathing in lateral position, 110
One-sided shoulder pull, 119
One sided stretch
    on stool, 120
    on table, 119
Orthopedic conditions, exercises in, 91-178
Osteoarthritis (*see* Arthritis)

Osteomyelitis of femur shaft, 160
Overstretching of muscles, 12, 22

P

Packs, hot, 61, 193
Pain, 55-68
   evaluation in case history, 67-68
   in fibrositis, 58
   heat in, 61-62
   histamine iontophoresis in, 66
   motor chain in, 66
   novocaine iontophoresis in, 64
   principles of treatment, 61
   reflex, 17
   rest, 25
   surface anesthetics in, 62-67
   in tension, 58-60
   tetanizing current in, 67
   triggerpoints of (see Triggerpoints)
Palpation, in back pain, 126
Palsy
   Bell's, 185
   cerebral, 201-212
      breathing exercises in, 225
      relaxation in, 51
Paralysis
   deltoid muscle, 183
   facial nerve, 185-186
   flaccid, 12
   of legs, 198
   medial nerve, 185
   peroneal nerve, 187
   radial nerve, 184-185
   sciatic nerve, 186
   spastic, 204-209
   ulnar nerve, 185
Paraplegia, 198
Passive exercises, 40
   assistive, 41
   relaxed, 40
   stretch, 24, 41
Patella, fractured, 161-162
Pectoral muscles, 219, 222
   elasticity of, 103, 108
   stretch of, 113
Pelvis
   angle, 102, 107
   tilt exercise, 127

Pendulum exercises, 48
Peripheral nerve lesions, 183-188
Peroneal nerve paralysis, 187
Poliomyelitis, 191-197
   breathing exercises in, 195, 223-224
Positioning exercises, 25, 44
   for strength-building, 47
Posture, 99, 100
   childhood patterns of, 83
   exercises for, 109
      breathing exercises with, 222-223
   functional measurements, 103-104, 108
   reflexes, 24-25
   strength and holding power measurements, 104-107
   structural measurements, 101-103, 107
Pregnancy, exercises in, 235
Prescription for exercises, 69-76
   supportive, 77-87
Procaine (see Novocaine)
Pseudo-hypertrophy of muscle, 12, 189
Psoas-iliacus strength building, 121-122
Pulmonary conditions, breathing exercises in, 225-228
Push-up exercise, 113

Q

Quadriceps strengthening, 154
Quadriplegia, spastic, 204

R

Radial nerve paralysis, 184-185
Radius fracture, at distal end, 149
Reflex relaxation, 41, 48
Reflexes
   conditioned, 25
   postural, 24-25
Regional function tests, 38
Relaxation, 18-20
   against gravity, 50
   concentric, 19
   by contrast, 50

by deconcentration, 50
eccentric, 19
exercises
  indirect, 238
  progressive, 237-238
  regional, 238
general training in, 48-50
isometric, 19
reflex, 41, 48
in rigidity, 23
in spasm, 23
in spastic paralysis, 205
in spasticity, 23
in tenseness, 23
Resistive exercise, 41
Respiration, 218-228 *(see also* Breathing)
Rest pain, 25
Rigidity, 22, 212
  relaxation in, 23
Rocking horse exercise, 114
Rotation, back, exercises for, 114-115
Rowing, effects of, 86
Running, injury from, 85, 157

S

Sandbag
  balance exercise, 117
  drop exercise, 113
  lift exercise, 113
Scalenus muscles, 219, 222
Scaphoid bone injuries, 150
Scapula
  distance from spine, 101, 107
  level of, 101, 107
  pull exercise, 113
Sciatic nerve lesions, 186-187
Sclerosis, multiple, 199-200
Scoliosis
  breathing exercises in, 223
  exercises for, 117-123
Serratus muscles, 219, 222
  exercise for, 113, 119
Shift exercise, in scoliosis, 118
Shoes, 78, 176
Shoulder
  acute injury of, 138-140
  bursitis of, 143-145
  circle exercise, 113
  dislocation of, 142-143
  exercises for, 113-114
  muscle injuries of, 146
  one-sided pull exercise, 119
  pull-up and hold-up exercise, 119
Sinusoidal current, 67
  in back pain, 132
  in neck injuries, 135
Sitting up exercise, 111, 128
Skating, effects of, 86
Ski-walking, 205
Skiing, injury from, 86
Sleeping
  habits, effects of, 79
  position, in upper extremity pain, 137-138
Spasm, 20
  grading of, 35
  in poliomyelitis, 193
  relaxation in, 23
  (see also Pain)
Spastic conditions
  hemiplegia, 214-216
  paralysis, 204-209
Spasticity, 21, 180-181
  grading of, 35
  relaxation in, 23, 50
  from upper motor neuron lesion, 56
Spinal cord lesions, 191-200
Spine
  cervical, 135-137
  fracture, 99, 125, 133-135
Sports, injury from, 83-86
Sprains, 96
  of ankle, 170-173
  of fingers, 151
  of knee joint, 163-166
  of wrist, 150
Spring, working against, 47
Statue exercise in scoliosis, 121
Stockings, tight, 78
Stomach balloon exercise, 111
Strain, 96-98
  of calf muscles, 169
  of hip muscles, 157-159
  in neck region, 135
  of shoulder muscles, 146
  of thigh muscles, 157-159

Strength, 5
  exercises for, 13-18, 45-47
    in back pain, 127-129
    in poliomyelitis, 192
    for quadriceps, 154
    for tibial muscle, anterior, 174
    for vastus medialis, 167
    for zero cerebral muscles, 206
  of muscles, 8-24, 181-182
    development of, 13-18
    measurement of, 31-33, 104, 108
    pathology of, 12-13
    physiology of, 8-11
  relative, 38
Stretching
  in back pain, 129-132
  in contracture, 23-24
  of gastrocnemius soleus, 110
  passive, 24, 42
  pectoral, 113
  in poliomyelitis, 195
  in scoliosis, 118
  standing, 110, 116
  wall stretch, 117
Substitution of muscles, 51
Surgery, breathing exercises after, 227-228, 234
Swimming, injury from, 85

T

Tabes dorsalis, 200-201
Tennis, injury from, 85, 147
  relaxation in, 23
Tenseness, 22
Tension
  athetoid, 211
  exercises for, 236-239
  gauging of, 36
  and neck conditions, 136
  pain in, 58-60
  relaxation training in, 48-50
  residual, 24, 36
  (see also Contraction)
Test
  of exercise tolerance, 232
  of muscles, 23-39, 125-126, 193
Tetanizing current, 67
  in back pain, 132
  in neck injuries, 135
Thigh muscle injuries
  acute, 157-159
  chronic, 159
Tibia fractures
  of condyles, 168
  of shaft, 168
Tibial muscle, anterior, strengthening of, 174
Tip-up exercise, 110
Toe touch exercise, 115
Torticollis, congenital, 136-137
Track and field, injury in, 85
Traction, 48
  in neck pain, 136
Transsection of spinal cord, 197
Trauma, exercise after, 91-178
Triggerpoints of pain, 57-58, 60
  in back pain, 133
  ethyl chloride spray in, 64
  in forearm pain, 148
  in hip pain, 155
  injection of, 98
  in neck pain, 136
  palpating for, 126
  in shoulder pain, 144, 145
  in spastic muscles, 199
Trunk, exercises for, 113-114
Twisters, use of, 204

U

Ulnar nerve paralysis, 185
Upper extremity, 137-152

V

Vastus medialis strengthening, 167
Vertebral fractures, 99, 125, 133-135

W

Walkers, use of, 205, 210
Wall stretch exercise, 117
Warm-up, 18, 158
  lack of, effects of, 32, 35
Weights
  carrying of, 48

lifting of, 32, 46, 165
Whiplash injuries, 135
Windmill exercise, 115
Wing spread exercise, 113
Working hazards, 81-82
Wrist
   acute injury to, 150
   chronic conditions of, 150
Wry neck, 136-137

Z

Zero cerebral muscles, 12, 16
   strengthening of, 206